Elizabeth Cook

KETO FOR WOMEN OVER 50

Keto for Women Over 50:
The Ultimate Guide of Keto Diet to Lose Weight Quickly and Lead a Healthy Lifestyle. Tasty and Healthy Recipes Simple to Prepare. 30-Day Meal Plan

© Copyright 2020 - All rights reserved.

Table of Contents

Introduction

The ketogenic diet is a popular diet with high levels of fat, sufficient proteins and low carbohydrates and is commonly called the ketogenic diet. It is called a low carbohydrate (LCHF) diet and a low carbohydrate diet. It was primarily developed for the treatment of epilepsy, which did not react to medication for diseases.

The diet was initially published in 1921 by Dr. Russell Wilder in the Mayo Clinic. Dr. Wilder found that fast epileptic patient deployment helped to reduce symptom frequency. At the time of its publication, there were few other options for treating epilepsy.

The ketogenic diet was widely used in the treatment of epilepsy in both children and adults for the next several decades. About 50 percent of patients reported at least a 50 percent reduction in seizures in several epilepsy studies.

However, in the 1940s and later, the arrival of anticonvulsant drugs relegated the ketogenic diet to an "alternative" medicine. It was much easier to use the pills compared to adhering to the strict ketogenic diet for the majority of health care providers as well as patients. It was subsequently ignored by most specialists in the treatment of epilepsy.

Hollywood producer Jim Abrahams sparked a renewed interest in the ketogenic diet in 1993. Abraham brought his 2-year-old son, Charlie, for epilepsy treatment at Johns Hopkins Hospital. Within days of using the ketogenic diet, Charlie experienced rapid seizure control.

In 1994, the Charlie Foundation was created by Jim Abrahams, which helped revive research efforts. His production of the TV film "First Do No Harm," starring Meryl Streep, also helped to promote the ketogenic diet significantly.

The meals were designed to give the body the right amount of protein for the growth and repair it needs. The calculation of the number of calories consumed was carried out to provide adequate amounts that could support and maintain the proper weight necessary for the height and weight of the child.

In principle, the ketogenic diet is a way to recalibrate the metabolism, through which you force the body to replace carbohydrates with fats in food and the body as an energy source. Once glucose sources have been depleted, the liver converts both food fat and body fat deposits into ketone and fatty acids, which it uses as an energy source for cells.

The Keto diet is an extremely effective method to lose weight quickly and effectively eliminate fat deposits from the body, without losing muscle mass, as long as it is applied properly.

Chapter One:
What Is the Keto Diet?

n the body, the carbohydrates consumed are transformed into glucose, which is carried to the cells by the blood and used as a source of energy. The goal of the ketogenic diet is to produce glucose, not the main energy source of the body, but body fat.

The basis of the ketogenic diet is to eliminate the body's sources of carbohydrates, forcing you to use the stock of fat tissue as an energy resource, maximising weight loss.

The name of this diet comes from the process of getting energy from the liver's breakdown of fat, generating ketone, which is then used instead of glucose to feed the body. This process of metabolism is called ketosis.

It is necessary to reduce drastically the number of carbohydrates ingested for the diet to work. Only 5 to 10 percent of the body's energy comes from carbohydrates, 5 to 15 percent protein, and 80 to 90 percent fat in the classic ketogenic diet, originally used to treat seizure disorders.

In the meantime, men and women tend to consume about 50 per cent of calories in the form of carbohydrates on a regular diet. Modified for weight loss and athletic performance improvements, the ketogenic diet allows greater freedom in protein consumption, keeping only the restriction on carbohydrates from 20 percent to 30 percent of your total calories.

The 4 Types of a Ketogenic Diet

A strict ketogenic diet is extremely difficult to maintain because carbon shapes the entire biological life around us; it is difficult to resist consuming at least a few carbohydrates absolutely during the day. The carbs are also important for muscle function. This is why there are transient forms of the keto diet: those that aim to help the person reduce the number of carbohydrates while remaining appetizing. The key here is to experiment and find what works better for you rather than blindly following pre-made formulas.

- **The standard ketogenic diet (SKD).** This method of ketogenic diet essentially aims to limit carbohydrate consumption to 30 g per day and is intended for people who do not exercise regularly.

- **The Ketogenic Targeted Diet (TKD).** You do TKD because you eat carbs just before and after the workout. It's that simple—ideal for people who do mild exercise during the day.

- **Ketogenic Cyclic Regime (CKD).** This is where we become serious. CKD involves loading a lot of carbohydrates at specific times and then exercising to spend everything. Ideal for those who have or are elite athletes with rigorous fitness programs.

- **A strong diet is ketogenic in protein (HPKD).** A daily ketogenic diet in which carbohydrates and proteins are minimized. The HPKD seeks to raise muscle mass by a 60 percent fat diet, 35–40 percent protein, and 0–5 percent carbohydrate intake.

What Is Ketosis?

Ketosis is a metabolic process by which the body goes from consuming sugar to produce energy by consuming fat. All kinds of sweets containing processed sugar, as well as natural sugar sources (fruits, sweet vegetables, roots, honey, maple syrup, etc.) and flour and white potatoes are referred to when we say sugar.

The human body uses sugar as an essential source of energy, not using the fats it accumulates. Glucose is the lightest molecule that the body can transform and use as energy. So the body is prone to choose sugar at the expense of any other energy source. In the case of eating without any type of sugar, the body no longer has glucose to produce energy, and ketosis occurs when our liver metabolizes fatty acids (burns fat) in the absence of sugar, turning molecules into ketones. These ketones are released into the blood, so the body uses them to ensure its optimal energy level.

Our pancreas produces 2 antagonistic hormones: insulin and glucagon. Insulin is a storage hormone, and through it, the amount of glucose in the blood is reduced when its level is increased. Insulin facilitates the penetration of glucose into cells, to use it as energy and to turn excess glucose and store it in adipose tissue.

Glucagon has the role of raising blood sugar levels, being a catabolic hormone that facilitates burning.

Glucagon transforms complex molecules into simple molecules so that the body can use them as an energy source.

When we stop giving our body sugar, our pancreas decreases insulin production and increases glucagon production, thus facilitating fat burning.

The human body is very intelligent and needs a short time to adapt to the new metabolic state and learn where it gets its energy. It does not need sugar or carbohydrates but will burn ketones.

Among the benefits of ketosis are:

- Burning old fats, which we have been carrying in our body for years;

- A constant level of fat burning, which determines a constant level of energy in the body during the day, without having ups and downs as in the case of sugar consumption;

- Weight loss, because there is also the regulation of hormones that cause fat accumulation;

- Regulating blood sugar levels;

- We give our pancreas a break after years of putting it to work;

- Mental clarity;

- Reducing inflammation in the body, which causes most diseases that people face today.

Are We in Ketosis? The First Symptoms

After a couple of days, ketosis should begin.

To understand that the body has entered the state of ketosis, a urine test can be carried out with special strips or blood tests using blood ketones or respiration meters by measuring the number of ketones in the breath.

Then there are clear signs that can reveal that you are in ketosis:

- Exhaustion.

- Dry mouth and feeling of thirst.

- Increased diuresis.

- Acetone breath or sweat due to the presence of acetone.

- Decreased appetite.

Various Low Carb Diets

The ketogenic diet is mainly used to shed extra pounds: it only affects fat mass and can achieve good results in a short time.

The keto diet has different methods that can be distinguished in:

- High protein ketogenic drugs or the Atkins diet.

- Norm protein ketogenic or VLCKD diet used in cases of obesity.

- Normo-hyperproteic ketogen is used not for weight loss but for the treatment of drug-resistant epilepsy.

Ketogenic Diet: How to Get to Ketosis

The ketogenic diet is a nutritional scheme that can be summarized as follows

- Low in calories.

- Low percentage and absolute carbohydrate content (low-carb diet).

- High protein content.

- A high percentage of lipids.

For the keto diet to work, we must first induce ketosis: how?

The first step is to eliminate sources of carbohydrates, such as bread, pasta, potatoes and sugar-based products, as well as dairy products, legumes, orange and red fruits and vegetables from your daily diet.

Only meat, eggs and fish are allowed in the ketogenic diet. Dietary supplements based on vitamins and Omega 3 can be added.

It is essential to drink a lot of water, at least two litres a day.

Who Can Follow a Keto Diet and When Is It not Recommended?

Ketosis is a state in which we are forcing the body to act in an exceptional emergency. If a healthy diet consists of consuming a good variety of foods in a balanced way, prioritizing vegetables, fruits and legumes; it seems obvious that the keto diet has its risks and that it is not valid for everyone.

The whole body needs energy, including the heart and brain, which need it constantly and uninterruptedly. When the brain cannot obtain its normal fuel, glucose, it is also forced to resort to ketone bodies in exceptional ways, which cannot fail.

Also, in extreme situations of ketosis, ketoacidosis can occur: ketone bodies -acids- lower the pH level of the blood, causing it to be more acidic. And this negatively affects the organs, with consequences of varying severity: bad breath, headaches, kidney problems, nausea, dizziness, cramps and muscle weakness, even brain edema.

For people with metabolic diseases, thyroid, kidney, liver or pancreas problems, diabetics or patients with TCAs, the keto diet is not recommended. Similarly, it is not recommended to follow this diet in the long term, as it is very unbalanced. It would not be an adequate diet to maintain weight since it is not possible to achieve adherence, and it can cause a rebound effect.

A strict ketogenic diet should only be used for specific purposes under certain circumstances and, if possible, always supervised by a professional. Depending on those goals—to lose weight, lose fat or define muscle—it could be adapted to the specific circumstances of each individual.

Contraindications and Who Should Not Follow It

The ketogenic diet used against obesity almost always leads to excellent results in the loss of fat mass. A specialist must follow it; it is not a do-it-yourself diet.

It is known that this diet has different contraindications. What are the main contraindications of the Keto diet?

- Ketosis is considered a toxic condition for the body: the disposal of ketone bodies over normal quantities can cause kidney fatigue.

- Maintaining the state of ketosis throughout the treatment is difficult. It is enough to ingest only one prohibited food to compromise the state of ketosis and push the body to draw energy from sugars.

- Initially, the weight loss is evident, but it is very difficult to maintain the weight achieved. There is a high risk of regaining all the pounds lost when carbohydrates are introduced again. The post-diet is complex and the foods must be reintroduced into one's diet gradually. The maintenance period must be followed by a dietician.

- Ketosis can cause discomfort such as nausea, decreased appetite, dizziness, headache, fatigue, breathing difficulties, constipation, excessive diuresis, sweat and acetone breath.

- It is a diet that cannot be followed for long periods because it is not completely balanced and would damage health.

- It can cause hypoglycemia, hypercholesterolemia and hypotension. The patient must be checked in the medical center.

Intermittent Fasting and Keto

Intermittent fasting (IF) is a tool that accelerates the transition to nutritional ketosis by increasing ketone body production and is often associated with the ketogenic diet.

Intermittent fasting is comprised of eating within a specific feeding window rather than eating throughout the day. Everyone, whether aware of it or not, fasts intermittently from dinner to breakfast. There are many methods for intermittent fasting. Some individuals fast for 16–20 hour intervals every other day while others follow a fast 24-hour day. The 16/8 process in which you eat in an 8-hour window, followed by a 16-hour fasting window, is the most prevalent intermittent fasting variety.

Although this practice is different between individuals who follow a diet based on carbohydrates and individuals who follow a ketogenic diet, it is possible to combine intermittent fasting with any diet, bringing numerous advantages such as:

- Reduction of triglycerides and LDL cholesterol.

- A decrease in blood pressure.

- Reduced risk of cancer (the absence of sugar during the state of ketosis does not make the cancer cells survive).

- Increased cell turnover.

- Increased fat-burning state.

- Increased mental clarity and concentration.

- Improved hunger control.

- Improved blood sugar level.

- Improvement of cardio-vascular activity.

- Improvement of physical performance thanks to the increase of energy.

- Acceleration of the state of nutritional ketosis.

How Does Intermittent Fasting Work?

There are different ways to perform intermittent fasting, the most common being 16/8. That is, we fast for 16 hours and eat meals for the remaining 8 hours.

Those who follow the range 16–8 normally skip breakfast and eat the meals of the day between 12 and 20 to penalize the meals that are shared with family or colleagues.

Fasting Phase

During the hours of fasting, it is very important to stay well hydrated; you can drink water (still or sparkling), tea, herbal tea or coffee without sugar. If you follow a ketogenic diet, you can safely take magnesium, sodium and potassium supplements during these hours.

This is how much you can take to keep your body fasting. Technically, any food or drink that contains more than 50 kcal breaks the fast.

Meal Phase

In the window of 8 hours dedicated to meals of the day, prepare the dishes as usual according to the diet you follow. It is important not to overeat, but to eat foods with many nutrients.

Frequency

Intermittent fasting can be practised every day of the week, only on weekdays or only on holidays according to your needs and habits.

Intermittent Fasting and the Keto for Mental Health

Various mental health benefits may be provided by both intermittent fasting and the ketogenic diet. Both have been clinically shown to improve memory, improve mental clarity and concentration, as well as prevent neurological disorders such as Alzheimer's and epilepsy from developing. With a carbohydrate diet, glucose changes can cause energy levels to change. Your brain uses a more consistent fuel supply during ketosis: ketones from fat stores, leading to better productivity and psychological performance.

Whenever you have a constant, ketone-clean energy source, your brain works better. Other than that, ketones are more effective in protecting your brain. Studies reveal that ketone bodies may have antioxidant properties that protect brain cells from free radicals and oxidative stress. In a study of adults with impaired memory, the growth of BHB ketones in their blood helped improve cognition. Also, when you're having trouble staying focused, your hormones can be the cause.

There are two main neurotransmitters in your brain: glutamate and GABA. Glutamate can help you create new memories and make your brain cells interact with each other; what helps retain glutamate is GABA. It can cause brain cells to stop functioning and eventually perish if there is too much glutamate. GABA is there for glutamate control and slowing down. Glutamate reigns freely if GABA levels are reduced, and mental fog occurs. By turning excess glutamate into GABA, ketones stop cell damage. While ketones increase GABA and decrease glutamate, they help prevent damage to cells, prevent cell death and improve concentration.

Researchers believe intermittent fasting enhances memory, decreases oxidative stress and preserves learning skills. Since your cells are subjected to moderate strain during fasting, the higher cells adapt to the stress by improving their particular ability to cope with these circumstances as the weaker tissues die. This is very similar to the tension your body gets when you hit the gym.

Exercise is a kind of stress adapted by your body to enhance and become more powerful. This also applies to intermittent fasting: you will continue to benefit as long as you are still alternating between eating habits and fasting. Similarly, understanding that ketosis and intermittent fasting, due to the synergistic and protective effects of ketones, will help improve cognitive functioning.

Chapter Two:
Keto for Women Over 50

Throughout our trajectory, not only are our circumstances (work, family, couple) and the life we lead (schedules and customs) changed. There are also modifications in our interior. Some of these make it difficult for us to keep fit or lose weight if that is our goal. Therefore, today we will see what those changes that occur in our bodies from the 50s are and how to deal with them.

The Body's Changes at 50

Some changes that occur in your body after 50 are as follows; the culprits of keeping fit is such a complex matter:

A Decrease in Testosterone Levels

With the arrival of andropause, the hormone levels begin to be reduced gradually, affecting the functioning of our body. Moreover, since testosterone is one of the main hormones responsible for muscle production and toning, once its levels decline, the performance of, for example, sports training is diminished.

Of course, a decrease in testosterone can cause a significant loss of muscle mass.

If you think this may be happening to you, we invite you to check it out with this quick and simple test: Check your testosterone levels.

Metabolism Slowdown

From 40/50 years of age, our basal metabolism (minimum calories that the body requires and consumes to digest food, generate hormones, and other basic functions of the human body) is reduced. This means that, when at 20 years of age, a man of 1.90 and 80Kg of weight required a minimum of 2500Kcal, today he will not need more than 1500Kcal.

The problem is that, generally, at 50, we want to continue eating the same thing we ate before, which gives the body an excess of calories that we do not spend, and that inevitably translates into weight gain.

Reduction of Muscle Mass and Increased Fat

As we told you at the beginning, the decrease in testosterone levels causes a reduction in muscle mass and in parallel, fat increases. In this way, the metabolism decreases even more since we have a greater amount of fat and less active tissue (muscle, which in turn is the one that burns the most calories).

How to Keep Body Changes At 50

At this point, you probably think that after 50, it is almost impossible to maintain a healthy weight. But the reality is that the effects of age and body changes of 50 can be mitigated and even avoided completely if we follow some guidelines.

1. **Take care of your diet:** Following a diet rich in nutrients, antioxidants, and vitamins can help reduce the effects of time and severity.

2. **Train your body:** Performing exercises regularly, working strength, and activating the muscles can be a great way to reverse body changes from a certain age. Furthermore, it has been found that performing physical activity normally leads to testosterone development. If you are being cared for with a degree of hormone dysfunction, of course, exercise can always be a fantastic ally when it comes to achieving good outcomes.

3. **Try to have a proper rest:** Did you know that high-stress levels, in addition to causing anxiety, can make you fat? Therefore, among other reasons, getting a restful break is a key point in maintaining physical and mental fitness at any age.

4. **Visit a health professional:** Although you can find a lot of information on the Internet, the best thing you can do for your health is to visit a medical professional who performs some basic tests (the complete analysis, biometrics, electrocardiogram, etc.) and can assess your state as a whole before prescribing yourself No type of treatment.

Keto Diet Benefits for Women Over 50

- **Increased physical and mental energy**: As we age, energy levels can drop for a variety of biological and environmental reasons. Followers of the Keto Diet often witness a boost in strength and vitality. One of the reasons why this event occurs is because the body burns excess fat, which is synthesized into energy. Also, the systemic synthesis of ketones tends to increase brain power and stimulate cognitive functions such as concentration and memory.

- **Improved sleep**: As they age, people tend to sleep less. People on keto diets often gain more and tire more easily from their exercise programs. This event could result in longer and more successful periods of rest.

- **Metabolism**: Ageing individuals often have a slower metabolism than during their youth. People who follow a long-term diet on keto dieters experience greater regulation of blood sugar, which can increase their metabolism.

- **Weight loss**: The body sheds accumulated body fat, which could precipitate the loss of excess pounds for faster and more effective fat metabolism. Also, it is believed that members have a decreased appetite, which could lead to a reduction in their calorie intake.

Keeping the weight off is important, especially in adulthood, when they need fewer calories per day than when they are in their twenties or thirties. However, it is still important to get nutrient-dense foods for the elderly from this diet.

Since it is common for ageing adults to lose muscle and strength, a nutritionist may recommend a high protein ketogenic diet.

- **Protection against specific diseases**: People over 50 who follow a diet may reduce their risk of developing conditions such as diabetes, mental disorders such as Alzheimer's disease, various cardiovascular diseases, different types of cancer, Parkinson's disease, non-alcoholic fatty liver disease, and multiple sclerosis.

- **Ageing:** Ageing is considered by some to be the most important risk factor for human diseases. Reducing ageing is, therefore, the logical step to minimize these disease risk factors.

The good news, which extends from the technical description of the ketosis process presented earlier, shows the increase in the energy of young people. Due to the use of fat as a source of fuel, the body can go through a process in which it can misinterpret the mTOR signal is suppressed and a lack of glucose is evident, signalling that ageing may be slowed down.

In general, over the years, numerous studies have shown that calorie restriction can help slow ageing and even increase lifespan. With the ketogenic diet, it is possible, without reducing calories, to act on ageing. An intermittent fasting method used with the keto diet can also affect vascular ageing.

When a person is intermittently fasting or following a keto diet, BHB or beta-hydroxybutyrate is produced, which is believed to induce anti-ageing effects.

What You Can Eat

Compared to other types of diets, the ketogenic diet is not very restrictive in terms of the foods you can eat, the only exception being carbohydrates and carbohydrates. Below are two lists, one with the types of foods allowed and one with the types of foods prohibited in the standard keto diet.

Food Allowed

Specifically, the diet during the ketogenic diet should include foods high in fat, medium in protein and very low in carbohydrates.

So you are allowed to eat:

- Chicken, beef, pork, lamb, fish, sheep

- Eggs

- Dairy products

- Hazelnuts

- Almonds

- Nuts

- Coconut oil, other vegetable oils

- Other nuts and seeds

- Butter

- Fermented cream

- Vegetables and fruits with very low carbohydrate content

- Berries (for fibre content)

Prohibited Food

When it comes to foods you are not allowed to eat, the ketogenic diet is indeed very strict. In the list below, you will find all the types of foods forbidden in this diet:

- Salt and sugar

- Any sugar preparations—juices, cakes, sweets, etc.

- Flour products—pasta, bread, pastries

- Cereals

- Alcoholic beverages

- Fruit, with a few minor exceptions

- Vegetables with a high content of carbohydrates-potatoes, maize, beans

- Sausages and other processed-meat products

As for the proportions of daily fats, proteins and carbohydrates, they must be in the following values:

- 75–80% fat

- 15–20% protein

- 5% carbohydrates

As several calories, a minimum of 2,000 calories is recommended for women and 2,500 calories for men.

Ketogenic Diet for Diabetes

As a treatment for epilepsy, ketogenic diets have been in use since 1924 in paediatrics. One that is high in fat and low in carbs is a ketogenic (keto) diet. The ketogenic diet's design is to shift the metabolic fuel of the body from burning carbohydrates to fats. The body, with the keto diet, metabolises fat into energy instead of sugar. A by-product of that process is ketones.

Ketogenic diets have been used over the years for the treatment of diabetes. One justification was that, by reducing the intake of carbohydrates leading to lower blood sugar, it treats diabetes at its root cause, reducing the need for insulin that minimises insulin resistance and associated metabolic syndrome. A ketogenic diet can thus improve blood glucose (sugar) levels while reducing the need for insulin at the same time. This point of view presents keto diets to counteract the consumption of high carbohydrate foods as a much safer and more efficient plan than injecting insulin.

A keto diet is a very restrictive diet. For instance, in the classic keto diet, about 80% of caloric requirements are obtained from fat and 20% from proteins and carbohydrates. This is a marked departure from the norm where the body runs on energy from sugar derived from the digestion of carbohydrates. Still, the body is forced to use fat instead of severely restricting carbohydrates. Healthy food intake from beneficial fats such as coconut oil, grass-pastured butter, organic pastured eggs, avocado, salmon fish, cottage cheese, avocado, almond butter, and raw nuts (raw pecans and macadamia) is required for a ketogenic diet. Individuals avoid all bread, rice, potatoes, pasta, flour, starchy vegetables, and dairy on ketogenic diets. The diet requires supplementation and is low in vitamins, minerals, and nutrients.

For people with type 2 diabetes, the low carbohydrate diet is frequently recommended because carbohydrates turn to blood sugar that causes blood sugar to spike in large quantities. Thus, eating extra sugar-producing foods is like courting danger for a diabetic who already has high blood sugar. Some patients can experience reduced blood sugar by switching the focus from sugar to fat.

Changing the primary energy source of the body from carbohydrates to fat leaves ketones in the blood behind the fat metabolism byproduct. This can be dangerous for some diabetic patients, as ketone accumulation may create a risk of developing diabetic ketoacidosis (DKA). DKA is a medical emergency that requires a physician's immediate care. Signs of DKA include consistently high blood sugar, dry mouth, polyuria, nausea, fruit-like odour in breathing, and difficulty breathing. A diabetic coma can lead to complications.

Chapter Three:
FAQ on Keto Diet

F ollowing a ketogenic diet can change your life, but such a diet can be frustrating and counterproductive if followed incorrectly. Here are some clarifications on the most burning questions regarding ketogenic diets.

Ketogenic diets are more popular than ever, but that doesn't mean they are even better understood by those who follow them. On the contrary, given the terms, styles of ketogenic diets and the purposes of each, there is more and more confusion.

Ketogenic diets can help anyone, whether they aim to lose weight, gain muscle mass or live a healthier life. Research on ketogenic diets has been conducted for decades and yet fascinating things are still being discovered about them.

The Terms "Fat-Adapted," "Ketosis Adaptation," and "Ketosis" Are Often Confused. Do They Mean The Same Things or Are There Differences?

Ketosis is induced when dietary carbohydrates are too low to be used as an energy source by the body, usually less than 50 grams per day. When this happens, it enters a unique metabolic state, a state in which the liver produces small organic molecules called ketone bodies in large enough quantities to give energy to the brain, organs and muscles. Thus, fat and these ketones are used as an energy source instead of carbohydrates.

Who has a typical western diet has ketone levels of 0.1–0.2 millimoles. But when consuming a truly ketogenic diet—75% fat, 20% protein and 5% carbohydrates—blood ketone levels increase to 0.5–5 millimoles, entering a state of nutritional ketosis. I know that ketosis levels vary a lot, but everyone's body and the response to the ketogenic diet also matter a lot.

Even when eating very good quality fats and rapidly depleting glycogen stores to enter ketosis in just a few days, there are still states of lethargy, fatigue and slowness. After two weeks, the body reaches maximum levels of ketones and, most importantly, regains energy, mental concentration and motivation. This turning point, when you completely adapt to the diet and which can last between two and 6 weeks, is called "ketosis adaptation."

Only when the body adapts to ketosis can it be said to have entered the metabolic state in which fat becomes the main source of energy. The process takes so long because the body's tissues need time to acquire the ability to oxidize (burn) fat for energy and use ketones. For example, the average amount of fat used during exercise is 30 grams per hour. After 6 weeks of adaptation to ketosis, the average increases to 90 grams per hour. From here, we can conclude that adaptation to ketosis is a term synonymous with adaptation to fat.

What Are the Mistakes Most Often Made by Those Who Follow a Ketogenic Diet?

The top 3 mistakes regarding the ketogenic diet are:

- Confusion of low-carb and ketogenic diets.

- Consumption of too much protein.

- Not enough time is left to adapt to ketosis.

Regarding the first two points, it must be understood that entering ketosis and increasing the concentration of ketones in the blood is essential to have a successful ketogenic diet. A baseline study by Dr. Young put students on diets with the same number of calories and protein, but with different carbohydrate intake (104 grams, 60 grams and 30 grams per day). They were all in a caloric deficit.

What happened was at least intriguing. In the group that consumed 104g of carbohydrates, 25% of the weight lost was in the form of muscle tissue, while those in the group that consumed 30 g of carbohydrates did not lose any muscle mass. The idea is that very low levels of carbohydrates are required to reach full ketosis. Ketones prevent the breakdown of amino acids such as leucine and thus preserve muscle mass.

It may seem like a good idea to eat a lot of protein. But a ketogenic diet is very high in fat, extremely low in carbohydrates and moderate in protein. When more than 1.5–1.8g/kilogram of body protein is consumed, they increase the formation of glucose, which makes it difficult to enter ketosis. Such a diet, very rich in fat and rich in protein, can negatively affect the development of muscle mass and muscle strength. So when you want to follow a ketogenic diet, resist the temptation to overdo it with protein!

It is equally important to have the patience to allow the body to adapt to the ketogenic diet. Most discontinue the diet before fully adapting to it. As it is known, in the first days of ketogenic diets, the physical performances decrease. But after the body adapts, you can have the same gains in muscle mass and strength as in a diet rich in carbohydrates but without the risk of gaining weight.

Doesn't Too Much Fat Upset Your Health? Is There Excess Fat When You Follow a Ketogenic Diet? How Do You Find the Balance Between Fat and Protein?

Yes, many studies link high-fat consumption to insulin resistance and obesity, high cholesterol, cardiovascular disease, fatty liver, etc. But an essential aspect must be understood; these studies are done on diets rich in fat and just as rich in carbohydrates!

This fateful combination is known as the "western diet" and leads to extremely many diseases. But research has shown that when there is only fat in the blood, they are used for energy. When there are fats in the blood at the same time as carbohydrates, fats are not used for energy (they are usually stored), and insulin resistance begins to manifest!

Why is this happening? Mainly because fats require a specific enzyme (CPT1) to be transported to the mitochondria (the place in cells where energy is created from macronutrients—fats, carbohydrates and proteins). High insulin levels reduce CPT1 levels and so fats are not transported to the mitochondria to be burned. In addition, as carbohydrates increase insulin levels a lot; it is easy to understand why the fat-carbohydrate combination is so unhappy. That is why, during a ketogenic diet, the consumption of carbohydrates must be extremely low in order not to prevent the transport and burning of fats. When these conditions are met, ketogenic diets have several health benefits, including lowering blood pressure, lowering triglycerides and cholesterol, and improving insulin sensitivity.

As for the balance between fat and protein, the secret is in choosing fatty meats. It can be a difficult idea for some to accept!

Very good sources of fatty foods to include in ketogenic diets are:

- Beef with a meat-fat ratio of 80/20.

- Salmon.

- Eggs.

- Salami and sausages (here the quality is extremely important; 95% of what you find in the barns are filthy, and the quality ones have prices to match - not for nothing a bad salami costs 20 lei and a quality one at the same amount costs 200 lei or more).

- Cream cheese.

- Bacon.

- Butter.

- Sour cream.

- Fatty oils such as nuts, cashews, and macadamia nuts.

If you want to eat lean meat or don't have anything else available, add some fat. Cook them in animal fat or butter. If you eat such foods, you will get the ideal proportion of fat/protein without bothering too much.

To all this can be added (it is even indicated) vegetables in moderate amounts, especially those with green leaves, such as salads, cabbage, mango, etc.

Does a Sad Meal Very Rich in Carbohydrates or a Cheated Day a Week Take You Out of Ketosis?

Many cannot conceive of following a ketogenic diet for a long time. That is why some variants of cyclic ketogenic diets have become very popular. Unfortunately, few of these have been studied in a clinical setting. The most well-known, such cyclic ketogenic diet is the one in which you follow a strict ketogenic diet for 5 days, and then you have 1–2 days of loading with carbohydrates.

There have also been studies comparing ketogenic diets with cliché ketogenic diets. It was found that although the subjects had the same caloric intake (usually those who follow the cliché ketogenic diet have a higher caloric intake when cheating—especially on weekends) and do the same exercise, they all lost the same number of pounds. Still, those who followed the ketogenic diet did not lose any muscle mass, while those who followed the cyclic ketogenic diet lost significant amounts of muscle mass. This is because cheating meals spoil your ketosis and practically a few days a week, you are in a semi-ketosis.

Moreover, muscle strength increases in those who follow the ketogenic diet, while those who follow the ketogenic diet, silica decreases. All are concrete indications that cycling takes you out of ketosis!

It seems that consuming very large amounts of carbohydrates after a long period of ketosis (10 weeks) leads to a large accumulation of fat in just one week. But if carbohydrates are gradually reintroduced into the diet, such as 1 gram per kilogram of body weight per week, there is no accumulation of fat.

This indicates that extreme fluctuations are not good, so the reintroduction of carbohydrates into the diet should be slow. A good method is the initial consumption of carbohydrates before training; they inhibit the insulin response. This method prevents fat burning during exercise, but it is a small sacrifice to succeed in maintaining the results obtained with the ketogenic diet. All these are general recommendations, and more research is needed in this area.

Are There More Effective Ways to Cycle Ketogenic Diets?

Not everyone can go on a ketogenic diet for long periods. They can follow a ketogenic diet for short periods several times a year with slow transitions from ketogenic diets to those with carbohydrates.

In 2013 such a study was done. Subjects followed a strict ketogenic diet for 20 days, followed by a 20-day transition period followed by a low-carb, high-protein diet. Then for 6 months, they had a Mediterranean diet, i.e. balanced in terms of protein, fat and carbohydrates. Then the subjects repeated the process.

It was found that the subjects burned fat at each ketone cycle and maintained their new body composition. Also, out of the 89 subjects, only 8 dropped out. So it has a very good adhesion rate.

What Does All This Tell Us?

Ketogenic diets can be very satisfactory in terms of physical performance and body composition (the ratio between fat and muscle mass). Using a ketogenic diet, you can burn a lot of fat and, at the same time, preserve your muscle mass, or you can increase your muscle mass without gaining weight.

But you have to be very dedicated to the diet, without cheated meals and leaks! Any escape takes you out of ketosis and pulls you back a lot.

It is important to experiment, especially if you want to refill with carbohydrates from time to time and monitor your ketosis level constantly. Invest in ketone urine tests (such as Ketostix) and test your ketosis regularly.

And finally, don't forget that at the end of the ketogenic diet, you have a transition period to a richer one in carbohydrates; don't do this suddenly.

Chapter Four:
The Best (Light) Exercises to Lose Weight for Women Over 50

I f you are over 50 years old, you will see that your body is starting to change. Losing weight is not as easy as before, and you start to feel pain in areas of your body that you have not noticed before. Your mood is fluctuating, too. What can you do to minimise the consequences of something as inevitable as having a birthday? Eat better, exercise, and seek out activities that stimulate the mind and body.

Why Do You Have to Exercise?

According to the Higher Sports Council, physical exercise is not only good for losing weight. It is necessary for other aspects of life.

- Increases muscle capacity, aerobic endurance, balance, joint mobility, flexibility, agility, coordination, etc.

- It has favourable effects on metabolism, regulation of blood pressure and prevention of obesity.

- It reduces the risk of suffering from cardiovascular diseases, osteoporosis, diabetes, and some types of cancer.

- It contributes to reducing depression, anxiety, improving mood and the ability to carry out life activities.

- It favours the establishment of interpersonal relationships (when done in a group, although in these moments of confinement, this is not possible) and social networks.

Why Do I Get Fatter With Age?

As we said, if you are over 50 (even if you are already in your 40s), you will have verified that getting rid of those extra kilos becomes an almost impossible mission. On the other hand, you have to make great sacrifices for it.

It's not that age makes you fat. But it is true that when we get older, it becomes more difficult to lose weight.

Energy expenditure at rest decreases approximately 5% every decade and, after 50, 10%, according to experts from Medical Option. This means that by consuming the same calories, your body will tend to store more and, therefore, you will gain weight more easily.

On the other hand, due to the hormonal decline that occurs in menopause, there are more tendencies to gain weight. This is due to the imbalance that exists between the drop in estrogen and progesterone. Progesterone is lost faster than estrogen, which is a hormone that tends to produce fat cells that progesterone counteracts.

Finally, our mobility and endurance, when we turn our birthday, is not the same as in our younger days. But we can fix it. For this reason, here are some exercises that you can do after 50 to lose weight and feel much better.

1. **Aerobic exercises:** Walking is an excellent exercise to lose weight, as long as you know how to walk well to lose weight, and it is also an aerobic exercise that makes you fit, activates your heart, and regulates your hormones. Ideally, you should walk an hour a day through different terrain and do intervals of greater intensity. If you feel like it and your physical shape is optimal, you can launch yourself into bigger strides or even jog.

2. **Squats:** they are as simple to practice, as they are difficult to do well. For this reason, to begin with, we suggest that you stand behind a chair and make the gesture of trying to sit down, with your legs spread across the width of your hips and your arms raised. It is a good way to activate the heart. Do it 10 times, rest and repeat three sets.

3. **Arm exercises:** The sagging of the inner part of the arms is something that worries many women and inevitable when we turn our birthday if we do not do exercises to tone the arms. What can you do? A very easy exercise: pass a towel or an elastic band behind your back and hold one end at the height of the buttocks with the left hand and the other at the height of the men. Stretch your right arm up and then your left arm down. Imagine, for example, that you are drying your back with a towel. Another way to work the arms, in addition to the abdomen, is to perform push-ups with a chair. Put it against the wall to prevent it from sliding. Perform six to eight repetitions depending on your fitness level.

4. **Back exercises:** Another exercise that you should do every day is that of the cat and the cow, a very simple way to relax your back and avoid pain. It is as simple as getting on all fours and mimicking the arch of the back just like a feline does. Do a counter-position and stretch your chest.

5. **Firm glutes:** If you are lucky enough to have stairs at home, go up and down them. It is a perfect aerobic exercise that will also work your glutes. Another way to work them is to do this exercise, called a bridge, and you can do it on a chair. Put your feet on it and try to lift your hips. Hold several breaths and go down slowly. If you feel safer, you can do it on the floor. And to increase the intensity, try lifting one leg and then the other. Hold several breaths and repeat five times on each leg.

6. **Irons to strengthen the abdomen:** Abs is no longer in fashion. Now, to strengthen the abdomen and reduce the waist, it is recommended to do other types of exercises such as planks. If you are a beginner, it is best to do them on a chair. And if you prefer to do other types of exercises, take note of those that the Sakuma method offers you. With them, you can reduce your waistline in just one month with gentle and simple exercises.

Chapter Five:
Breakfast Recipes

Omelette Caprese

Total time: 5 minutes.

Servings: 2 portions.

Ingredients

- 2 tablespoons olive oil

- 6 eggs

- 100 grams cherry tomatoes, cut in halves or tomatoes cut into slices

- 1 tablespoon fresh basil or dried basil

- 150 grams (325 milliliters) fresh mozzarella cheese

- Salt and pepper

Preparation

1. Break the eggs in a bowl to mix and add salt and black pepper to taste.

2. Beat well with a fork until everything is completely mixed.

3. Add basil and stir.

4. Cut the tomatoes into halves or slices.

5. Chop or slice the cheese. Heat the oil in a large skillet.

6. Fry the tomatoes for a few minutes.

7. Pour the egg mixture over the tomatoes.

8. Wait until it becomes a little firm and add the cheese.

9. Lower the heat and let the omelet harden.

10. Serve immediately and enjoy it!

Nutrition

- **Net carbohydrates:** 3% (4g)

- **Fiber:** 1g

- **Fats: 73%** (45g)

- **Protein: 24%** (33g)

- **Kcal:** 560

Scrambled Eggs

Total time: 5 minutes.

Servings: 1 portion.

Ingredients

- 2 eggs
- 30 grams butter
- Salt and ground black pepper

Preparation

1. Using a fork, beat the eggs along with some salt and pepper. Over medium heat, melt the butter in a nonstick skillet. Look carefully: butter is not turning golden! Pour the eggs into the pan and mix until they are creamy and cooked a little less than you like, for 1–2 minutes.

2. Remember that even once you put them on your plate, the eggs will continue to cook.

3. These creamy eggs pair well with many low carb dishes that are popular. Of course, classic accompaniments such as bacon or sausage may be eaten. Still, other great options are available, such as salmon, avocado, cold cuts and cheese (cheddar, fresh mozzarella or feta). If you are really hungry (or if you are cooking big eggs), do not be shy: use more butter!

Nutrition

- **Net carbohydrates:** 1% (1g)
- **Fiber:** 0g **Fat:** 85% (31g)
- **Protein:** 14% (11g)
- **Kcal:** 327

Keto Eggs with Avocado and Bacon Candles

Total time: 12 minutes.

Servings: 4 portions.

Ingredients

- 2 eggs, hard

- ½ avocado

- 1 teaspoon olive oil

- 60 grams bacon

- Salt and pepper

Preparation

1. Preheat the oven to 180–200°C (350°F).

2. Put the eggs in a pot and cover with water.

3. Bring to a boil and let simmer for 8–10 minutes.

4. Place the eggs in ice water as soon as they are made to make it easier to peel them.

5. Split the eggs into two halves along and take out the yolks.

6. Put them in a small bowl. Add avocado and oil to the bowl and mash until mixed—salt and pepper to taste. Place the bacon on a baking sheet and bake until crispy. Take 5–7 minutes. You can also fry them in a pan.

7. With a spoon, carefully add the mixture to the egg whites and place the bacon candle. Enjoy it!

Nutrition

- **Net carbohydrates:** 2% (1g) **Fiber:** 2g **Fat:** 83% (13g) **Protein:** 15% (5g) **Kcal:** 144

Asparagus and Artichoke Salad with Dijon Vinaigrette

Total time: 2 hours and 10 minutes.

Servings: 6 portions.

Ingredients

- 1 cup asparagus spears, cooked
- 1 cup artichoke hearts, cooked
- 1 egg, hard-boiled, chopped finely
- 1 tablespoon thyme, chopped
- 2 garlic cloves, minced
- 2 tablespoons chicken stock, reduced-sodium
- 1 tablespoon cider vinegar
- 1 tablespoon Dijon mustard
- 1 teaspoon dry mustard
- 1 tablespoon flat-leaf parsley, minced
- 1/4 teaspoon salt
- Freshly ground pepper
- 4 teaspoons olive oil
- Green bean

Preparation

1. Arrange the cooked asparagus, artichoke hearts and green beans on a platter.

2. Put the vinegar, broth, dry mustard, Dijon mustard, pepper, thyme, salt and garlic, in a blender or food processor. Stir the mixture over the veggies.

3. Put parsley and egg on top of your salad.

4. Cover with plastic wrap and put in the fridge for at least 8 hours.

5. Leave at room temperature for half an hour before serving.

Nutrition

- **Net carbohydrates:** 3% (4g)

- **Fiber:** 1g

- **Fats:** 73% (45g)

- **Protein:** 24% (33g)

- **Kcal:** 560

Romanesco Salad with Quail Eggs

Total time: 5 minutes.

Servings: 6 portions.

Ingredients

- 1 avocado, mashed

- 12 pieces quail eggs, hard-boiled, halved

- 2 green Romanesco salad tomatoes, chopped

- 1 raw egg yolk

- 2 red Romanesco salad tomatoes, chopped

- 1 lemon, freshly squeezed

- Pinch of sea salt

- Pinch of white pepper, to taste

Preparation

1. Combine avocado, egg yolk, and lemon juice in a bowl; season well with salt and pepper. Place the remaining ingredients into a salad bowl. Drizzle in the avocado-lemon mix. Toss salad to combine. Serve.

Nutrition

- **Net carbohydrates:** 1% (1g)

- **Fiber:** 0g

- **Fat:** 85% (31g)

- **Protein:** 14% (11g)

- **Kcal:** 327

Cucumber Jicama Salad with Cashew Butter

Total time: 10 minutes.

Servings: 4 portions.

Ingredients

For Salad

- 1 jicama, sliced into ¼-inch thick matchsticks

- 1 celery stalk, julienned

- 2 cucumbers, sliced into ¼-inch thick matchsticks

- Pinch of sea salt - Pinch of black pepper, to taste

- 4 tablespoon cashew butter

For cashew butter

- 1 cup cashew nuts, toasted, cooled before processing, Pinch of sea salt

- 1 tablespoon coconut oil, melted

Preparation

For salad

1. Toss ingredients into the salad bowl to combine. Chill for 15 minutes before serving.

For cashew butter

2. Place the ingredients in a blender with cashew butter. Process until smooth, often scraping down the blender's sides.

Nutrition

- **Net carbohydrates:** 1% (1g) **Fiber:** 0g **Fat:** 85% (31g) **Protein:** 14% (11g) **Kcal:** 327

Apple Bruschetta with Almonds and Blackberries

Total time: 50 minutes.

Servings: 5 portions.

Ingredients

- 1 apple, sliced into ¼-inch thick half-moons

- ¼ cup blackberries, thawed, lightly mashed

- ½ teaspoon fresh lemon juice

- ⅛ cup almond slivers, toasted

- Sea salt

Preparation

1. Drizzle lemon juice on apple slices. Place these on a tray lined with parchment paper. Spread a small number of mashed berries on top of each slice. Top them up with the desired amount of almond slivers. Sprinkle sea salt on the "bruschetta" just before serving.

Nutrition

- **Net carbohydrates:** 4% (9g)

- **Fiber:** 14g

- **Fat:** 84% (75g)

- **Protein:** 12% (24g)

- **Kcal:** 820

Fried Vegetable Brown Rice

Total time: 15 minutes.

Servings: 4 portions.

Ingredients

- 4 cups brown rice, cooked
- 1 ½ cups carrots, diced
- ¾ cup celery, diced
- 1 ½ cup green onions, chopped
- 1 ½ tablespoon garlic, minced
- ¾ cup red bell pepper, diced
- 3 tablespoon fresh chillies, minced
- 3 tablespoon fresh cilantro, chopped
- 1 red bell pepper, diced
- 1 ½ tablespoon soy sauce
- 3 teaspoon sesame oil
- Ground white pepper, to taste
- 3 tablespoon olive oil

Preparation

1. Place the wok over a high flame and heat it.
2. Add the vegetable oil and swirl to coat.
3. Stir in the shallots, garlic, and chillies until fragrant, then add the carrots and reduce to medium flame. Sauté until crisp-tender.

4. Stir in the rice, celery, and bell pepper and mix well.

5. Pour in the soy sauce and season with salt and white pepper.

6. Stir until the rice is decomposes and heats up.

7. Fold in the cilantro and transfer to a serving dish.

8. Drizzle with sesame oil and serve right away.

Nutrition

- **Net carbohydrates:** 1% (1g)

- **Fiber:** 0g

- **Fat:** 85% (31g)

- **Protein:** 14% (11g)

Breakfast Arroz Caldo

Total time: 50 minutes.

Servings: 5 portions.

Ingredients

- 6 eggs, white only

- 1½ cups brown rice, cooked

For the filling

- ¼ cup raisins

- ½ cup frozen peas, thawed

- 1 white onion, minced

- 1 garlic clove, minced - Oil, for greasing

Preparation

1. For the filling, spray a small amount of oil into a skillet set over medium heat.

2. Add the onion and garlic. Stir until the former is limp and transparent. Stir-fry while breaking the clumps, about 2 minutes. Add the remaining ingredients; stir-fry for another minute. Turn down the heat, and let filling cook for 10 to 15 minutes, or until juices are greatly reduced. Stir often. Turn off the heat.

3. Divide into 6 equal portions. For the eggs, spray a small amount of oil into a smaller skillet set over medium heat. Cook eggs. Discard yolk; transfer to holding the plate. To serve, place 1 portion of rice on a plate, along with 1 portion of filling and 1 egg white. Serve warm.

Nutrition

- **Net carbohydrates:** 3% (4g) **Fiber:** 1g **Fats:** 73% (45g) **Protein:** 24% (33g)

- **Kcal:** 560

Cooled Almond Soup

Total time: 10 minutes.

Servings: 4 portions.

Ingredients

- 2 garlic cloves, sliced

- 4 slices bread, crust removed

- 5 teaspoons apple cider vinegar

- 1 cup blanched almonds

- 3 cups chilled water

- 5 tablespoons olive oil

For garnish

- Toasted flaked almonds

- Grapes, seedless

Preparation

1. Break bread in a bowl. Pour over chilled water. Leave for 5 minutes. Combine almonds and garlic in a blender. Process until finely ground. Add the soaked bread. Process until smooth.

2. Gradually put the oil until the mixture forms a smooth paste.

3. Add sherry vinegar and the remaining chilled water. Process until smooth. Season with salt and pepper. Chill in the fridge for 3 hours.

4. Ladle the soup into a chilled bowl. Scatter with almonds and grapes. Serve.

Nutrition

- **Net carbohydrates:** 2% (1g) **Fiber:** 0g **Fat:** 84% (31g) **Protein:** 15% (12g) **Kcal:** 329

Couscous with Lettuce and Carrots Salad

Total time: 20 minutes.

Servings: 3 portions.

Ingredients

- 1 cup couscous

- 2 carrots, diagonally sliced

- 2 cups baby romaine lettuce

- 1 tablespoon flaxseed oil

- ¼ teaspoon ground coriander

- 1/8 teaspoon smoked paprika

- 2 tablespoons lime juice

- 1 red bell pepper, chopped

- ¼ teaspoon ground cumin

- 4 cups water

- 1 tablespoon extra-virgin olive oil

- Pinch of salt, add more if needed

- Pinch of pepper; add more if needed

Preparation

1. Pour 5 cups of water into a large saucepan.

2. Bring to a boil. Add couscous.

3. Reduce heat to low. Cover and allow simmering for 10 minutes. Stir occasionally.

4. Drain and rinse under cold water.

5. Meanwhile, in a mixing bowl, combine flaxseed oil, olive oil coriander, cumin, paprika, and lime juice.

6. Whisk the mixture well. Stir in red bell pepper and carrots. Season with salt and pepper.

7. Toss well to coat. To serve, line a salad plate with lettuce.

8. Top an equal amount of the salad.

Nutrition

- **Net carbohydrates:** 3% (4g)

- **Fiber:** 1g

- **Fats:** 73% (45g)

- **Protein:** 24% (33g)

- **Kcal:** 560

Nutty Oats Pudding

Total time: 5 minutes.

Servings: 3–5 portions.

Ingredients

- ¼ cup rolled oats

- 1 tablespoon yoghurt, fat-free

- 1 ½ tablespoon natural peanut butter

- ¼ cup dry milk

- 1 teaspoon peanuts, finely chopped

- ½ cup water

Preparation

1. Use a microwaveable-safe bowl. put together peanut butter and dry milk. Whisk well.

2. Add water to achieve a smooth consistency.

3. Add oats; cover the bowl with plastic wrap.

4. Create a small hole for the steam to escape.

5. Place inside the microwave oven for 1 minute on high powder.

6. Continue heating, this time on medium power for 90 seconds.

7. Let sit for 5 minutes. To serve, spoon an equal amount of cereals in a bowl top with peanuts and yoghurt.

Nutrition

- **Net carbohydrates:** 2% (1g)**Fiber:** 0g **Fat:** 84% (31g) **Protein:** 15% (12g) **Kcal:** 329

Cranberry and Raisins Granola

Total time: 35 minutes.

Servings: 4 portions.

Ingredients

- 4 cups old-fashioned rolled oats

- 1/4 cup sesame seeds

- 1 cup dried cranberries

- 1 cup golden raisins

- 1/8 teaspoon nutmeg

- 2 tablespoons olive oil

- 1/2 cup almonds, slivered

- 2 tablespoons warm water

- 1 teaspoon vanilla extract

- 1 teaspoon cinnamon

- 1/4 teaspoon salt

- 6 tablespoons maple syrup

- 1/3 cup honey

Preparation

1. In a bowl, mix the sesame seeds, nutmeg, almonds, oats, salt, and cinnamon. In another bowl, mix the oil, water, vanilla, honey and syrup.

2. Gradually pour the mixture into the oats mixture.

3. Toss to combine. Spread the mixture into a greased jellyroll pan. Bake in a preheated oven at 325° F for 55 minutes.

4. Stir and break the clumps every 10 minutes. Once you get it from the oven, stir the cranberries and raisins. Allow cooling.

5. This will last for a week when stored in an airtight container and up to a month when stored in the fridge.

Nutrition

- **Net carbohydrates:** 1% (1g)

- **Fat:** 85% (31g)

- **Protein:** 14% (11g)

- **Kcal:** 327

Breakfast Omelette

Total Time: 10 minutes.

Servings: 2 portions.

Ingredients

- 2 eggs

- 3 egg whites

- 1 tablespoon water

- 1/2 teaspoon olive oil

- 1/4 teaspoon salt

- ¼ teaspoon ground pepper

Preparation

1. In a bowl, beat the eggs, egg whites, salt, pepper and water, until frothy. Heat half of the oil in a skillet over medium heat. Pour half of the egg mixture. Cook for a couple of minutes while lifting the edges using a spatula every once in a while. Fold into a half. Turn the heat to low and continue cooking for a minute. Repeat the process for the rest of the egg mixture.

Nutrition

- **Net carbohydrates:** 1% (1g)

- **Fiber:** 0g

- **Fat:** 85% (31g)

- **Protein:** 14% (11g)

- **Kcal:** 327

Breakfast Marinated Egg

Total time: 12 minutes.

Servings: 4 portions.

Ingredients

- 6, soft-cooked eggs, peeled, cooled

For marinade

- ½ cup brown sugar

- ½ cup mirin

- 1 cup water

- 1 cup sake

- ½ cup tamari

Preparation

1. Combine the marinade ingredients in a bowl. Stir until sugar dissolves. Place eggs into an airtight non-reactive container just small enough to fit all these in. Pour in the marinade. Eggs should be completely submerged in liquid. Discard leftover marinade, if any. Line the container's rim with generous layers of saran wrap. Secure the container lid. Chill the eggs for 24 hours before use. Drain well after. Discard marinade. Pat dry before eating, using, or storing away.

Nutrition

- **Net carbohydrates:** 3% (4g)

- **Fiber:** 1g **Fats:** 73% (45g)

- **Protein:** 24% (33g) **Kcal:** 560

Crispy Cheese Keto Omelette

Total time: 20 minutes.

Servings: 4 portions.

Ingredients

Omelet

- 2 eggs

- 2 tablespoon whipping cream

- Salt and ground black pepper

- 1 tablespoon butter or coconut oil

- 75 grams grated or sliced cheese, cured

Filling

- 2 sliced mushrooms

- 2 sliced cherry tomatoes

- 2 tablespoon (30g) cream cheese

- 15 grams spinach sprouts

- 30 grams turkey cold cuts

- 1 teaspoon dried oregano

Instructions

1. In a bowl, beat the eggs, cream, salt, and pepper.

2. Heat a tablespoon of butter in a nonstick skillet over medium heat. Spread the cheese evenly in the pan so that it covers the entire bottom. Fry over medium heat until bubbly.

3. Carefully incorporate the egg mixture over the cheese and reduce heat. Cook a few minutes without stirring.

4. Fill half with mushrooms, tomatoes, spinach, cream cheese, turkey, and oregano. Fry a few more minutes.

5. When the egg mixture begins to set (it can still be quite loose on top, but not too much) turn the empty half over half with the ingredients, forming a half-moon. Fry a few more minutes and enjoy!

Nutritional value

- **Calories** 520

- **Fat** 46g

- **Saturated** fat 28g

- **Sodium** 692mg

- **Carbohydrates** 10g

- **Fibe** 5g

- **Sugar** 13g

- **Protein** 116g

Chapter Six:
Lunch Recipes

Watermelon and Tomato Soup with Parmesan

Total time: 30 minutes.

Servings: 4 portions.

Ingredients

- 500 grams watermelon pulp (seedless)

- 650 grams ripe cherry tomatoes

- 5 grams basil (1 handful)

- 2 tablespoon white wine vinegar

- 5 tablespoon olive oil

- Salt

- Pepper

- 125 grams mozzarella (45% fat in dry matter)

- 30 grams pine nuts (2 tablespoons)

- 50 grams parmesan in one piece (30% fat in dry matter)

Preparation

1. Cut the watermelon pulp into small pieces and place in a blender.

2. Wash the cherry tomatoes and set aside about 8 pieces.

3. Wash the basil, shake dry and put a few leaves aside.

4. Put the rest of the basil with stems and the rest of the tomatoes in the blender.

5. Add vinegar and 4 tablespoons of oil, season with salt and pepper and puree everything as finely as possible. Then pass through a fine sieve into a bowl and cool for about 1 hour.

6. In the meantime, cut the mozzarella into small cubes; roast pine nuts in a hot pan without fat over medium heat for 3 minutes.

7. Set aside cherry tomatoes in slices, cut aside basil leaves into fine strips. Mix the mozzarella cubes, tomato slices, pine nuts, and basil strips with the remaining oil in a bowl.

8. To serve, fill the chilled soup into bowls, top with the mozzarella mixture and grate the parmesan.

Nutrition

- **Calories:** 359kcal (17%)

- **Protein:** 14g (14%)

- **Fat:** 27g (23%)

- **Carbohydrates:** 16g (11%)

- **Added sugars:** 0g (0%)

- **Fiber:** 3g (10%)

Baked Eggplant Salad

Total time: 35 minutes.

Servings: 4 portions.

Ingredients

- 3 eggplants

- 1 green pepper

- 1 red bell pepper

- 1 yellow pepper

- 1 large onion

- 1/2 cup olive oil

- 1/4 cup vinegar

- 3 tablespoons chopped black olives

- 2 cloves (large) minced garlic

- 1 bay leaf

- 2 tablespoons oregano

- 2 tablespoons chopped parsley

- Salt to taste

Instructions

1. Remove some of the eggplant's peel, cut into thin slices lengthwise and then cut into strips.

2. Soak the sliced eggplants in salted water for half an hour, then rinse the salt and squeeze.

3. Cut the onion and bell pepper into strips, put in a baking dish, and add the eggplant, garlic, bay leaf, parsley, oregano, olive, and salt.

4. Drizzle with half the vinegar and bake in a medium preheated oven for 45 minutes. Remove from oven and drizzle with olive oil and remaining vinegar.

5. Let cool and serve.

Nutrition

- **Calories:** 114.4kcal

- **Protein:** 0.7g (1%)

- **Carbohydrates:** 5.2g (2%)

- **Fat:** 10.3g (16%)

- **Cholesterol**

- **Sodium:** 183.2mg (7%)

- **Cholesterol** 0mg (0%)

Microwave Quick Keto Bread

Total time: 2 minutes.

Servings: 1 portion.

Ingredients

- 3 tablespoons almond flour
- ½ teaspoon phylum powder
- ½ teaspoon baking powder
- A pinch of salt
- 1 large egg
- butter

Preparation

1. Add the dry ingredients to a small bowl, then butter and egg.
2. Mix well. Lubricate the microwave, mug, or small bowl, and add the butter.
3. Put the bread in the microwave for 80–100 seconds. Gently place the bread on a cutting board and cut in half.

Nutrition

- **Calories:** 220kcal **Carbohydrates:** 4g
- **Proteins:** 4g **Fat:** 21g
- **Saturated fat:** 7g **Cholesterol:** 33mg
- **Fiber:** 2g
- **Sugar:** 0g

Chick Curry (Thai Chicken)

Total time: 28 minutes.

Servings: 4 portions.

Ingredients

- 2 skinless, boneless chicken breasts (not too small)
- 3 tablespoons olive oil
- 1 small onion, finely chopped
- 2 cloves garlic, minced
- 3 tablespoons curry powder
- 1 teaspoon ground cinnamon
- 1 teaspoon paprika
- 1 bay leaf
- 1/2 teaspoon freshly grated ginger root
- 1 tablespoon tomato extract
- 1 bottle coconut milk
- 1/2 lemon (juice)
- 1 red bell pepper
- 1 cup pineapple (optional)

Preparation

1. In a bowl, season the chicken cubes with salt and lemon juice and set aside.
2. Put in a pan, the olive oil, garlic, onion, and saute until golden brown.

3. Then put the chicken in the pan and saute until golden brown.

4. Add the pineapple (optional), curry, cinnamon, paprika, bay leaf, tomato extract, ginger, and red pepper.

5. Saute for a few more minutes (if necessary, add a cup of water).

6. Add coconut milk, cook for a few more minutes and serve.

Nutrition

- **Calories:** 383kcal (19%)

- **Carbohydrates:** 10g (3%)

- **Protein:** 29g (58%)

- **Fat:** 25g (38%)

Baked Fish Fillet

Total time: 25 minutes.

Servings: 4 portions.

Ingredients

- 500 grams fish fillet (tilapia, saint peter or other)

- 4 large potatoes peeled in 0.5 cm thick slices

- 2 chopped tomatoes

- 1/2 bell pepper (if it is large)

- 1 medium diced onion

- 1 tablespoon full of capers

- Green smell to taste

- Coriander to taste (optional)

- 1/2 tablespoon salt

- 1 clove garlic (small) well squeezed

- Olive oil to taste

Instructions

1. Season the fish fillet with salt and garlic and set aside.

2. Mix the tomatoes, onions, peppers, capers and season with a little salt and add the green and coriander smell. Reserve.

3. Grease a refractory with olive oil and line with the raw potatoes.

4. Cover the potatoes with the fish and spread over the tomato mixture.

5. Drizzle with plenty of olive oil and bake for about 30 to 40 minutes.

6. When you dry the liquid that accumulates in the bottom of the pan when it is baking and is golden brown is ready.

7. Serve with integral or white rice; it is delicious!

Nutrition

- **Calories:** 235kcal

- **Total Fat:** 16g

- **Cholesterol:** 110mg

- **Protein:** 23g

Chicken with Okra

Total time: 1 hour and 30 minutes.

Servings: 4 portions.

Ingredients

- 5 thighs

- 1 lemon juice

- 5 cloves minced garlic

- Salt to taste

- Black pepper to taste

- 1 + 1/4 cup oil

- 1 kilo chopped okra

- 1 chopped onion

- 2 bay leaves

- 2 tablespoon tomato sauce

- Green smell to taste

Instructions

1. Arrange the drumsticks on a platter and season with 1 lemon juice, garlic, salt, and black pepper to taste.

2. Cover the platter with plastic wrap and set aside in the refrigerator for 30 minutes; in a skillet, heat 1 cup of oil.

3. Add the okra and saute to drool out. Remove the okra and place it on a plate with paper towels to drain.

4. In another pan, heat 1/4 cup oil and fry the drumsticks. Remove the thighs and add the chopped onion and bay leaves to the pan, sauté well.

5. Return the drumsticks to the pan and add the tomato sauce.

6. Cover with hot water and cook for 20 minutes. Add the okra, the green smell and set the salt.

Nutrition

- **Calories:** 367kcal (17%)

- **Protein:** 16g (16%)

- **Fat:** 15g (13%)

- **Carbohydrates:** 42g (28%)

- **Added sugar:** 0g (0%)

- **Dietary fiber:** 7g (23%)

Mexican Baked Beans and Rice

Total time: 30 minutes.

Servings: 2 portions.

Ingredients

- 5 milliliters (1 teaspoon) unsalted butter

- 1 chopped yellow onion

- 3/4 cup (190 milliliters) basmati rice

- 5 milliliters (1 teaspoon) ground cumin

- 1 seeded jalapeno pepper

- 300 milliliters (1 1/4 cups) chicken stock

- 125 milliliters (1/2 cup) tomato sauce

- 3/4 cup (190 milliliters) canned black kidney beans

- 30 milliliters (2 tablespoons) finely chopped parsley

- 1 lime

- Salt and pepper to taste

Preparation

1. Melt the butter in a saucepan and add the onion. Simmer.

2. Add the ground cumin and rice. For approximately 2 minutes, continue cooking.

3. Add the pepper from the Jalapeno, with chicken stock and season, deglaze.

4. Add the tomato sauce, cover, and cook for about 12 minutes over medium heat.

5. Add the black beans and parsley when the rice is cooked.

6. Continue to cook for several minutes.

7. Add the lime juice, pepper, salt, and serve.

Nutrition

- **Calories:** 176kcal

- **Protein:** 4g

- **Fat:** 9g

- **Carbohydrates:** 19g

- **Added sugar:** 2.4g

- **Dietary fiber:** 1.8 g

Sea Bass and Peppers Salad

Total time: 20 minutes.

Servings: 3 portions.

Ingredients

- 150 grams fillet sea bass very clean

- 100 grams assorted lettuces

- Chives, to taste

- 1 fresh or roasted red pepper

- Cherry tomatoes to taste

- 1 garlic clove and parsley

- 1 leek

- 1 carrot

- 1 tablespoon olive oil

- Salt and lemon to taste

Directions

1. We put the fillet of sea bass in aluminum foil.

2. In the mortar, chop the garlic and parsley, add 2 small teaspoons of oil and cover the fillet of sea bass with it.

3. We also put some leek and carrot strips on the sea bass fillet (the vegetable ribbons can be made with the fruit peeler) and a little salt.

4. Now we close the foil tightly and take it into the oven at 120ºC for 8–10 minutes. Once cooked, let it cool.

5. In a salad bowl, we put the lettuce mixture, chop the chives and pepper very finely. We add it too.

6. Add the cherry tomatoes cut into quarters. Add only a small teaspoon of olive oil, salt, and lemon as a dressing, stir well, and now add the fish with the vegetables we have cooked in the oven and ready to eat.

Nutrition

- **Calories:** 633kcal (30%)

- **Protein:** 50g (51%)

- **Fat:** 25g (22%)

- **Carbohydrates:** 48g (32%)

- **Added sugar:** 0g (0%)

- **Dietary fiber:** 7.5g (25%)

Fish in Tomato Sauce

Total time: 45 minutes.

Servings: 4 portions.

Ingredients

- 4 frozen white fish fillets of your choice

- 2 cups cherry tomatoes cut in half

- 2 finely sliced garlic cloves

- 120 milliliters light chicken broth

- 60 milliliters dry white wine (or use more chicken stock)

- 1/2 teaspoon salt

- 1/2 teaspoon black pepper

- 1/4 cup finely chopped fresh basil leaves (to garnish)

Preparation

1. Place the tomatoes, garlic, salt, and pepper in a pan over medium heat. Cook for 5 minutes or until the tomatoes are soft.

2. Add chicken broth, white wine (if used), frozen fish fillets, and chopped basil. Cover and simmer 20–25 minutes, until the fish is fully cooked.

3. Finally, sprinkle with an additional handful of chopped basil and serve on a bed of rice, couscous or quinoa, if desired.

Nutrition

- **Calories:** 110kcal (5%) **Protein:** 2g (2%) **Fat:** 6g (5%)

- **Carbohydrates:** 12g (8%) **Added sugar:** 3.8g (15%) **Dietary fiber:** 1.1g (4%)

Exotic Tuna, Sauce and Rice

Total time: 10 minutes.

Servings: 3 portions.

Ingredients

- 1 can tuna

- 1 can pineapple slices

- 2 large onion

- 200 milliliters coconut milk

- 50 milliliters broth

- 1 tablespoon oil (peanut, sunflower, or sesame oil)

- 1/2 butter

- 1 tablespoon curry or curry paste, red

- 1 tablespoon flour

- Salt and pepper, whiter, ground

- 2 cups of rice

Preparation

1. The onions are first halved from top to bottom and then sliced lengthwise into thin slices and sautéed in oil and butter over low heat for 5 minutes.

2. Then the drained tuna is added and fried.

3. Mix the curry and flour, continue for a short time.

4. Add the broth and top up with the coconut milk.

5. Simmer briefly, add the sliced pineapple (two slices or to taste) and season with salt, pepper and a good dash of pineapple juice.

6. Serve with rice.

Nutrition

- **Calories:** 143kcal (7%)

- **Protein:** 9.8g (10%)

- **Fat:** 0.35g (0%)

- **Carbohydrate:** 27.21g (18%)

- **Added sugar:** 1.05g (4%)

- **Dietary fiber:** 4.35g (15%)

Custard with Quark and Fruit

Total time: 45 minutes.

Servings: 12 portions.

Ingredients

- 1000 milliliters milk - 6 tablespoon sugar

- 2 pack pudding powder, vanilla

- 1-kilo Quark (lean quark) - 4 tablespoon sugar

- 1 point vanilla sugar

- 250 milliliters milk

- 500 milliliters whipped cream

- 2 teaspoon vanilla sugar

- 1-kilo fruit of your choice (cherries, strawberries, peaches, etc.)

Preparation

1. Cook the custard according to the preparations; add the milk, sugar, and let it cool down. Cover it so that it does not form any skin. Mix the quark with the four tablespoons of sugar, the vanilla sugar and the 250 ml of milk. Beat the cream with the vanilla sugar until stiff.

2. Prepare fruit, corer according to variety, cut small. Once the pudding has cooled, stir in the cottage cheese. Then fold in the whipped cream and the fruit.

3. Again cold for a while and then enjoy!

Nutrition

- **Calories:** 256kcal (12%) **Protein:** 18g (18%) **Fat:** 15g (13%)

- **Carbohydrates:** 11g (7%) **Added sugar:** 0g (0%) **Dietary fibre:** 7g (23%)

All Seafood Stock

Total time: 1 hour and 35 minutes.

Servings: 3 portions.

Ingredients

- 2 pounds fresh lobster, shrimp peelings

- 8 cups water

- 1 carrot, chopped

- 1 tablespoon dried chilli flakes

- 2 pounds frozen fish heads and frames

- 2 large onions, halved

- 1 large celery rib, halved

- 1 garlic head, halved

- 2 tablespoon olive oil

- 1 tablespoon apple cider vinegar

- ¼ teaspoon white pepper

- 2 shallots

Preparation

1. Preheat the oven to 220°C or 425°F. Line a deep roasting pan with aluminium foil.

2. Place fish heads and frames into a roasting dish, along with garlic and shallots. Drizzle oil on top.

3. Place roasting pan into the middle rack of the oven; roast fish for 25 minutes. Remove pan from the oven.

4. Transfer contents into a slow cooker, along with the remaining ingredients. Secure lid. Cook broth for 8 hours.

5. Strain out and discard solids. Ladle portions into bowls. Serve with bread and salad of choice.

Nutrition

- **Calories:** 80kcal (4%)

- **Protein:** 2g (2%)

- **Fat:** 1g (1%)

- **Carbohydrates:** 14g (9%)

- **Added sugar:** 0g (0%)

- **Dietary fiber:** 1g (3%)

Pesto Chicken Sandwich

Total time: 1hour and 30 minutes.

Serving: 4 portions.

Ingredients

- 3 garlic cloves, chopped

- 1 cup fresh basil leaves

- 2 tablespoon pine nuts, freshly toasted

- Pinch of sea salt; add more if needed

- Pinch of black pepper, to taste

- 1/3 cup extra virgin olive oil

- 1/3 cup cashew cheese

- 4 pieces of bread, halved

- Olive oil, for brushing

- 2 cups chicken breast, cooked, shredded

- 2 cups arugula leaves

- 1 beefsteak tomato, sliced into thick medallions

- ¼ cup cashew cheese

Preparation

1. For the bread, lightly coat sides of the bread with olive oil. Toast in an oven toaster. Set aside.

2. For the pesto, put garlic cloves, basil leaves, pine nuts, salt, and black pepper into a blender.

3. Process several times until basil leaves are minced.

4. Pour olive oil and cashew cheese into the blender.

5. Process until the desired consistency is achieved.

6. Adjust taste if needed. To serve, put together shredded chicken and an equal amount of pesto in a bowl. Mix well.

7. Spread cashew cheese on toasted wheat bread; layer with arugula leaves, chicken, and tomato slices. Top it with the other bread slice. Serve.

Nutrition

- **Calories:** 80kcal (4%)

- **Protein:** 2g (2%)

- **Fat:** 1g (1%)

- **Carbohydrates:** 14g (9%)

- **Added sugar:** 0g (0%)

- **Dietary fiber:** 1g (3%)

Buttered Prawns in Garlic Rice

Total time: 25 minutes.

Servings: 2 portions.

Ingredients

- ½ cup cooked brown or wild

- 4 tiger prawns, shelled, deveined, halved lengthwise

- 1 garlic, minced

- ⅛ teaspoon butter

- ⅛ teaspoon olive oil

- Sea salt

Preparation

1. Pour the oil in a wok over high heat. Sauté butter until golden and aromatic. Do not burn. Remove from wok immediately.

2. In the same wok, stir-fry prawns until these turn coral, about 3 minutes. Season well. Add in the remaining ingredients, including garlic.

3. Cook until rice is well heated, about 3 more minutes. Serve warm.

Nutrition

- **Calories:** 80kcal (4%) **Protein:** 2g (2%)

- **Fat:** 1g (1%) **Carbohydrates:** 14g (9%)

- **Added sugar:** 0g (0%)

- **Dietary fiber:** 1g (3%)

Chapter Seven:
Recipes for Dinner

Fennel and Apple Gratin

Total time: 20 minutes.

Servings: 4 portions.

Ingredients

- 4 apples (Elstar)

- 200 milliliters white wine

- 2 teaspoons mustard seeds

- 1 teaspoon fennel seeds

- Salt

- 150 grams mountain cheese (e.g. south tyrolean stilfser)

- 1 small fennel bulb

- 1 tablespoon hazelnuts

Preparation

1. Rinse the apples, cut them in half and hollow out the core with a ball cutter. Simmer white wine with mustard seeds, fennel seeds and salt for 5 minutes.

2. Braise the apple halves in the wine brew until just about done. Lift the apples from the wine brew with a slotted spoon and place them on a baking dish. Pour in some brew.

3. Cut the mountain cheese into pieces and add to the apples. Gratin briefly under the preheated grill so that the cheese melts.

4. Clean, rinse and finely chop the fennel. Chop the hazelnuts.

5. Serve apples sprinkled with fennel and hazelnuts.

Nutrition

- **Calories:** 338kcal (16%)

- **Protein:** 13g (13%)

- **Fat:** 14g (12%)

- **Carbohydrates:** 31g (21%)

- **Added sugars:** 0g (0%)

- **Fiber:** 5.6g (19%)

Egg and Avocado Sandwich with Crab Salad

Total time: 25 minutes.

Servings: 4 portions.

Ingredients

- 2 eggs

- 1 organic lime

- 10 grams ginger

- 1 teaspoon honey

- 50 milliliters rapeseed oil

- 200 grams Greek yogurt

- Salt

- Cayenne pepper

- 200 milliliters North Sea crabs (ready to cook; pre-cooked)

- 1 avocado

- 100 milliliters radicchio

- 1 box shiso cress

- 8 slices whole-grain sandwich bread

Preparation

1. Boil eggs hard in boiling water in 8–9 minutes. Remove, quench under running cold water and peel.

2. While the eggs are boiling, rinse the hot lime, pat dry, and rub the skin. Halve the lime and squeeze out the juice.

3. Peel and finely grate the ginger. Puree the lime zest, 1-teaspoon lime juice, ginger, honey, oil, and yogurt; season with salt and cayenne pepper.

4. Fold in the crab. Halve the avocado, remove the stones, lift the pulp from the skin and cut into fine slices.

5. Drizzle with a little lime juice. Wash the radicchio, shake it dry and remove the leaves from the stalk. Slice the eggs. Cut the cress from the bed. Toast slices of bread. Cover 4 slices with eggs, crab salad, avocado, radicchio, and cress and cover with 1 slice of bread each.

6. Halve sandwiches and arrange on plates.

Nutrition

- **Calories:** 458kcal (22%)

- **Protein:** 20g (20%)

- **Fat:** 29g (25%)

- **Carbohydrates:** 29g (19%)

- **Added sugar:** 0g (0%)

- **Dietary fiber:** 7.3g (24%)

Low Carb Tomato Soup

Total time: 50 minutes.

Servings: 4 portions.

Ingredients

- 1 organic lemon

- 300 grams yogurt (0.3% fat)

- Salt

- Pepper

- 200 grams vegetable onion (1 vegetable onion)

- 2 garlic cloves

- 4 stems basil

- 1600 grams peeled tomatoes (2 can)

- 1 tablespoon olive oil

- 700 milliliters vegetable broth

- 125 milliliters soy cream

Preparation

1. Rinse lemon with hot water, rub dry and finely grate the peel. Mix with yoghurt, a little salt and pepper in a bowl.

2. Let the yoghurt drain for several hours—preferably overnight—in a sieve lined with a coffee filter bag. Peel the onion and garlic.

3. Finely dice the onion. Chop the garlic. Wash the basil, shake dry, pluck the leaves from 1 stem and set aside.

4. Mash tomatoes in a can or a bowl; heat olive oil in a pot. Sauté the onion and garlic over medium heat while stirring.

5. Add the tomatoes and 3 basil stalks, fill with the stock and bring to the boil. Cook on medium heat for 20 minutes.

6. Remove the basil and puree the soup very finely. Add soy cream to the soup and bring to the boil again.

7. Season to taste with salt and pepper. Put the tomato soup on a plate, spread the lemon yogurt over it and garnish everything with the basil leaves.

Nutrition

- **Calories:** 193kcal (9%)

- **Protein:** 8g (8%)

- **Fat:** 9g (8%)

- **Carbohydrates:** 18g (12%)

- **Added sugars:** 0g (0%)

- **Fiber:** 6.4g (21%)

KETO FOR WOMEN OVER 50

Mediterranean Vegetables

Total time: 15 minutes.

Servings: 4 portions.

Ingredients

- 2 small zucchinis - 1 small eggplant
- 1 yellow pepper - 1 red pepper
- 3 tomatoes
- 1 onion
- 1 clove of garlic
- 4 tablespoon olive oil
- Salt
- Pepper from the mill

Preparation

1. Clean, wash, slice the zucchini. Wash the eggplant, cut in slices, quarter-long. Clean, wash, and dice peppers.

2. Wash tomatoes, cut into cubes. Peel and dice garlic and onion; heat olive oil in a medium-heat pan. Fry the garlic, onions and peppers, occasionally turning over medium heat for about 5 minutes.

3. Add zucchini and eggplant and cook for 5–7 minutes; salt and pepper season. Add the tomatoes and cook 2–3 minutes.

Nutrition

- **Calories:** 170kcal (80%) **Protein:** 5g (5%) **Fat:** 11g (9%) **Carbohydrates:** 12g (8%)
- **Added sugars:** 0g (0%) **Fiber:** 6.6g (22%)

90 | P a g .

Cod the Portuguese Way

Total time: 20 minutes.

Servings: 4 portions.

Ingredients

- 5 cooked potatoes approx. 600g

- 2 onions

- 4 cod fillets without skin, 150g each

- Olive oil for the mold

- 1 clove of garlic

- 1 red pepper

- 60 grams green olives without stones

- 4 tomatoes

- Salt

- Pepper from the mill

- 100 milliliters dry white wine

- 30 milliliters olive oil

Preparation

1. Peel the potatoes and cut into slices. Peel the onions and cut lengthways into fine strips. Wash the cod and pat dry with kitchen paper.

2. Brush a baking dish with olive oil. Peel and chop the garlic and sprinkle in the pan. Layer the potatoes on top.

3. Wash the pepper, cut in half, clean and cut into small cubes, cut the olives into slices. Wash and slice the tomatoes.

4. Preheat the oven to 180–200°C top and bottom heat. Spread the tomato slices on the potatoes, season with salt and pepper.

5. Layer the fish on top, salt, pepper and sprinkle with onion, paprika and olives. Pour the white wine and drizzle the contents of the baking dish with the olive oil.

6. Cook in the oven for about 25 minutes.

Nutrition

- **Calories:** 445kcal (21%)

- **Protein:** 40g (41%)

- **Fat:** 18g (16%)

- **Carbohydrates:** 25g (17%)

- **Added sugars:** 0g (0%)

- **Fiber:** 4.3g (14%)

Pumpkin Gratin with Leek and Hazelnuts

Total time: 20 minutes.

Servings: 4 portions.

Ingredients

- 1 kilo Hokkaido pumpkin

- 2 poles leek

- 10 grams butter (2 teaspoons; room temperature)

- 200 milliliters vegetable broth

- Salt

- Chilli flakes

- 2 branches rosemary

- 125 grams mozzarella (1 scoop)

- 60 grams hazelnuts

Preparation

1. Wash the pumpkin, cut in half, remove the seeds and cut the pulp into narrow wedges.

2. Clean the leek, cut in half lengthways, wash and cut into pieces approx. 8 cm long. Brush one large or 4 small baking dishes with butter.

3. Put the pumpkin and leek in the pan, pour in the stock and season with salt and chilli flakes.

4. Wash the rosemary, shake it and cut finely. Sprinkle over the vegetables.

5. Cut the mozzarella into strips. Roughly, chop the nuts.

6. Sprinkle both over the vegetables and bake the gratin in a preheated oven at 160°C (fan oven 140°C; gas: level 2) for about 30 minutes.

Nutrition

- **Calories:** 294kcal (14%)

- **Protein:** 13g (13%)

- **Fat:** 19g (16%)

- **Carbohydrates:** 17g (11%)

- **Added sugars:** 0g (0%)

- **Fiber:** 9.3g (31%)

Vegetable Frittata with Pumpkin

Total time: 10 minutes.

Servings: 4 portions.

Ingredients

- 350 grams pumpkin pulp (e.g., from nutmeg or Hokkaido pumpkin)

- 30 grams butter (2 tablespoons)

- 1 tablespoon white wine vinegar

- Salt

- Pepper

- 1 pole leek

- 150 grams broccoli florets

- 3 branches thyme

- 100 grams feta

- 50 grams manchego (1 piece)

- 8 eggs

- 50 grams crème Fraiche cheese

Preparation

1. Dice the pumpkin. Heat the butter in a pan. Add pumpkin and fry for 2 minutes over medium heat.

2. Deglaze with vinegar and 50 ml water, season with salt, pepper and cook covered for approx. 5 minutes.

3. Wash and clean the leek and cut into fine rings. Wash the broccoli and drain well.

4. Mix the leek and broccoli with the pumpkin and cook briefly until the liquid has evaporated.

5. In the meantime, wash the thyme, shake dry and finely chop the leaves. Dice the feta and grate the Manchego.

6. Whisk the eggs with the crème Fraiche, salt, pepper and thyme. Mix the feta and manchego. Pour over the vegetables.

7. Allow to bake briefly and bake in a preheated oven at 180°C (convection 160°C; gas: level 2–3) for about 15 minutes. Let slide out of the pan and serve cut into pieces.

Nutrition

- **Calories:** 393kcal (19%)

- **Protein:** 23g (23%)

- **Fat:** 29g (25%)

- **Carbohydrates:** 9g (6%)

- **Added sugars:** 0g (0%)

- **Fiber:** 4.1g (14%)

Vegans Sliced À La Bombay

Total time: 25minutes.

Servings: 2 portions.

Ingredients

- 100 grams vegan roast piece (brand "Wheaty")

- 75 grams parboiled Rice

- 100 grams broccoli

- 150 grams pineapple

- 1/4 onion

- 100 milliliters coconut milk

- Some Curry, pepper and vegetable broth

- Maybe some Locust bean gum

Preparation

1. Cook the rice, chop the vegan roast and sauté.

2. For the sauce, fry the onion and deglaze with coconut milk.

3. Add the broccoli and cook. Season the sauce with curry, pepper and some vegetable stock (if the sauce is too liquid, you can use some carob seed flour). In the end, add the pieces of pineapple (unsweetened) to the sauce.

Nutrition

- **Calories:** 680kcal **Fat:** 19g

- **Carbohydrates:** 78g **Protein:** 44g

Summery Bowls with Fresh Vegetables and Protein Quark

Total time: 10 minutes.

Servings: 2 portions.

Ingredients

- 100 grams green salad

- 100 grams radish

- 200 grams kohlrabi

- 70 grams carrots

- 70 grams red lentils

- 50 grams tomatoes

- 2 spring onions

- 20 grams nuts/seeds

- 150 grams soy yogurt

- 2 tablespoon mixed herbs

- 1 teaspoon lemon juice

- 20 grams Nutri-Plus Shape & Shake, neutral

- 1 pinch salt, pepper

Preparation

1. Wash the salad and the vegetables and peel the kohlrabi. Simmer the red lentils for about 7 minutes. In time, cut/grate the vegetables.

2. Mix the soy yogurt with the lemon juice, the protein powder, some salt/pepper, and the herbs.

3. Arrange all the ingredients together on a deep plate or bowl and top with the spring onions and nuts/seeds.

Nutrition

- **Calories:** 550kcal

- **Carbohydrates:** 90g

- **Fat:** 9g

- **Protein:** 38g

Baked Turkey Breast with Cranberry Sauce

Total time : 2hrs

Serving 6

Ingredients

- 2 kilos of whole turkey breast

- 1 tablespoon olive oil

- 1/4 cup onion

- 2 cloves of garlic

- Thyme

- Poultry seasonings

- Coarse-grained salt

- 2 butter spoons

- 1/4 cup minced shallot

- 1/4 cup chopped onion

- 1 clove garlic

- 2 tablespoons flour

- 1(1/2) cups of blueberries

- 2 cups apple cider

- 2 tablespoons maple honey

- Peppers

Preparation

1. Grind in the blender ¼-cup onion, 2 garlic with herbs. Add 1 tablespoon of oil and spread the breast with this.

2. Put on the baking tray, add a cup of citron and bake at 350ºF (180°C) so that the thermometer records 165ºF (75°C) inside, about an hour, add ½ cup of water if necessary.

3. Bring the citron to a boil, add the blueberries, and leave a few minutes. In the butter (2 tablespoons), add the onion (1/4 cup), shallot, and garlic (1 clove).

4. Add the flour to the onion and shallot and leave a few minutes. Add the citron, cranberries, and honey and leave on low heat. Season with salt and pepper, let the blueberries are soft, go to the processor, and if you want to strain.

5. Return to the fire and let it thicken slightly.

6. Slice the thin turkey breast and serve with the blueberry sauce.

Nutritional value

- **Calories:** 604 kcal

- **Carbohydrate:** 57 g

- **Fat:** 13 g

- **Protein:** 66 g

- **Cholesterol:** 184 mg

- **Sodium:** 839 mg

- **Potassium:** 954 mg

- **Fiber:** 4g

- **Calcium:** 75mg

Zucchini Noodles with Avocado Cream and Tomatoes

Total time: 10 minutes.

Servings: 2 portions.

Ingredients

- 400 grams zucchini

- 1 avocado

- 100 grams cherry tomatoes

- 10 grams sesame

- 5 grams olive oil

- 1 clove of garlic

- 2–3 stems basil

- 1 pinch each salt and pepper

Preparation

1. Cut the zucchini into the pasta with a spiral cutter or peeler. Peel a garlic clove and add it to the avocado along with the olive oil and some basil.

2. Puree the ingredients to a creamy mass. Quarter the cherry tomatoes and put them under the avocado cream; season with salt and pepper and mix with the zucchini noodles.

3. Sprinkle with sesame and enjoy

Tip: If you do not tolerate raw zucchini so well, you can fry them briefly in a pan.

Nutrition

- **Calories:** 450kcal **Carbohydrates:** 15g

- **Protein:** 10g **Fat:** 35g

Gluten-Free Chickpea Soup with Nutri-Plus Shape & Shake

Total time: 20 minutes.

Servings: 1 portion.

Ingredients

- 1 red onion

- 2 garlic cloves

- 500 grams sweet potatoes

- 400 grams chickpeas, cooked

- 1 centimeter ginger

- 1 vegetable stock

- 30 grams Nutri-Plus neutral protein powder, gluten-free

- 1 teaspoon salt

- 1 teaspoon pepper

- 1 teaspoon turmeric

- 1 teaspoon nutmeg

- 1 teaspoon coconut oil

Preparation

1. First, remove the shell from the onion, garlic, and ginger, slice it into thick slices, and fry it in a little coconut oil. Peel the sweet potato and cut it into large pieces.

2. Once the onions are glassy, you can put the sweet potato in the pot. Stew everything together and then extinguishes it with the vegetable broth.

3. Let it simmer for about 10–12 minutes until the sweet potato is tender enough, then add the chickpeas.

103 | P a g .

4. Let everything simmer for another 5 minutes. Get the soup off the stove. Then take a blender and puree the soup a bit.

5. Now add the protein powder and let the blender do the rest of the work. Mix the soup until no pieces are left.

6. Season with the spices and enjoy. If you like, then you can roast some chickpeas and add to the soup as a topping.

Nutrition

- **Calories:** 550kcal

- **Carbohydrates:** 90g

- **Fat:** 9g

- **Protein:** 38g

Chapter Eight:
Recipes of Sweets and Snacks

Eggplant and Chickpea Bites

Total time: 50 minutes;

Servings: 6

Ingredients

- 3 large eggplant cut in half (make a few cuts in the flesh with a knife)

- Spray oil

- 2 large cloves garlic, peeled and deglazed

- 2 tablespoon coriander powder

- 2 tablespoon cumin seeds

- 400 grams canned chickpeas, rinsed and drained

- 2 tablespoon chickpea flour

- Zest and juice of 1/2 lemon

- 1/2 lemon quartered for serving

- 3 tablespoon polenta

Preparation

1. Heat the oven to 200ºC (180ºC rotating heat, gas level 6). Spray the eggplant halves generously with oil and place them on the meat side up on a baking sheet. Sprinkle with coriander and cumin seeds, and then place the cloves of

garlic on the plate. Season and roast for 40 minutes until the flesh of eggplant is completely tender. Reserve and let cool a little.

2. Scrape the flesh of the eggplant in a bowl with a spatula and throw the skins in the compost. Thoroughly scrape and make sure to incorporate spices and crushed roasted garlic. Add chickpeas, chickpea flour, zest, and lemon juice. Crush roughly and mix well; check to season. Do not worry if the mixture seems a bit soft—it will firm up in the fridge.

3. Form about twenty pellets and place them on a baking sheet covered with parchment paper. Let stand in the fridge for at least 30 minutes.

4. Preheat oven to 180ºC (rotating heat 160ºC, gas level 4). Remove the meatballs from the fridge and coat them by rolling them in the polenta. Place them back on the baking sheet and spray a little oil on each. Roast for 20 minutes until golden and crisp. Serve with lemon wedges. You can also serve these dumplings with a spicy yogurt dip with harissa, this delicious but spicy mashed paste of hot peppers and spices from the Maghreb.

Nutritional value

*   **Calories:** 72 g

*   **Protein**: 3 g

*   **Carbohydrates:** 18 g

*   **Dietary fiber**: 4 g

*   **Total fat:** 1 g

*   **Sodium:** 63 mg

*   **Phosphorus:** 36 mg

*   **Potassium:** 162 mg

Parmesan Cheese "Potatoes"

Total time 20mins

Serving 6

Ingredients

- 75 grams grated Parmesan cheese

- 1 tablespoon (8 grams) Chia seeds

- 2 tablespoon (20 grams) whole flaxseeds

- 2½ tablespoon (20 grams) pumpkin seeds

Instructions

1. Preheat the oven to 180–200°C (350°F).

2. Cover a baking sheet with baking paper.

3. Mix the cheese and seeds in a bowl.

4. With a spoon, put small piles of the mixture on the baking paper, leaving some space between them. Do not flatten the piles. Bake for 8 to 10 minutes checks frequently. The "potatoes" should take a light brown color, but not dark brown.

5. Remove from the oven, let cool before removing the "potatoes" from the paper, and serve them.

Nutritional value

- **Calories:** 383kcal

- **Carbohydrates:** 10g

- **Protein:** 29g

- **Fat:** 25g

Chili Cheese Chicken with Crispy and Delicious Cabbage Salad

Total time 40 mins

Serving 4

Ingredients

Chili Cheese Chicken

- 400 grams chicken

- 200 grams tomatoes

- 100 grams cream cheese

- 125 grams cheddar

- 40 grams jalapenos

- 60 grams bacon

Crispy Cabbage Salad

- 0.5 pcs casserole

- 200 grams Brussels sprouts

- 50 Grams of almonds

- 3 paragraph mandarins

- 1 tablespoon olive oil

- 1 teaspoon apple cider vinegar

- 0.5 teaspoon salt

- 0.25 teaspoon pepper

- 1 tablespoon lemon

Preparation

1. Turn on the oven at 200°C. Cut tomatoes in half and place in the bottom of a dish. Put chicken fillets in the dish, place half of the cream cheese on each chicken fillet and sprinkle with cheddar. Spread jalapenos in the dish and bake it first for 25 minutes. Place bacon on a baking sheet with baking paper, and bake it for 10 minutes. Next, make the cabbage salad. When the chicken dish has been given 35 minutes, it should be done.

2. Put the Brussels sprouts and cumin in a food processor and blend it well and thoroughly. Make the dressing of juice from one mandarin, olive oil, apple cider vinegar, salt, pepper, and lemon juice.

3. Put the cabbage in a dish and spread the dressing over. Chop almonds, cut the tangerine into slices and place it on the salad.

4. Sprinkle the bacon over the chicken dish before serving, and serve it with the cabbage salad!

Nutritional value

- **Calories** 367

- **Fat** 19.7g

- **Cholesterol** 87mg

- **Sodium** 1830mg

- **Carbohydrate** 10.4g

- **Protein** 36.8g

Keto Pumpkin Pie for Halloween, Sweet, and Spicy

Total time 50mins

Serving 2

Ingredients

Pie Bottom

- 110 grams almond flour

- 50 grams sucrine

- 0.5 teaspoon salt

- 1 tsp. of protein powder

- 1 paragraph eggs

- 80 grams butter

- 15 grams fiber

The Filling

- 1 pcs Hokkaido pumpkin

- 3 paragraph egg yolks

- 60 milliliters coconut milk the fat, not the water

- 1 teaspoon vanilla powder

- 15 grams protein powder

- 1 teaspoon cinnamon

- 50 Grams of sucrine

- 0.5 teaspoon black cardamom

- 0.5 teaspoon cloves

Preparation

1. Preheat oven to 175°C. Start making the bottom, as it needs to be baked!

2. Mix all the dry ingredients in a bowl and add the wet ones. Stir it well and control with your hands so you can shape it into a lump. Take a piece of baking paper and place the dough lump. Place a piece of baking paper on top and flatten the dough. Shape it to the size of a regular pie mold with a diameter of 24cm. Use a rolling pin if necessary. Prick holes in the bottom and behind the dough and place in the oven for 8–10 minutes. Be careful about giving it too much (we did it the first time).

3. Then make the filling. Cut the meat from your Hokkaido (or the garbage of the meat!) and cook it in a saucepan for 15–20 minutes. Put it in a food processor and add all the other ingredients and blend it well.

4. Pour the stuffing into the baked pie and bake again for approx. 25–30 minutes more until it looks golden and done. Eat when cooled or cool down first. A dollop of whipped cream is great too!

Nutritional value

- **Calories:** 143kcal

- **Carbohydrates:** 3g

- **Protein:** 5g

- **Fat:** 13g

Sweet Potato Pie

Total time 2hrs

Serving 4

Ingredients

- 250 grams wheat flour type 1700

- 2 tablespoon whole cane sugar

- 125 grams butter

- Salt

- 600 grams sweet potatoes

- 4 eggs

- 100 milliliters whipped cream

- 2 tablespoon maple syrup

- 2 teaspoon cinnamon

Preparation

1. Knead flour, 1 tablespoon of whole cane sugar, pieces of butter, 1 pinch of salt and 1–2 tablespoons of cold water first with the dough hook of the hand mixer, then with your hands form a smooth dough.

2. Roll out the dough between 2 layers of cling film (approx. 30cm Ø) and place in a greased tart or spring-loaded pan (24cm), forming a 3cm high edge. Chill for 30 minutes.

3. In the meantime, wash the sweet potatoes and boil them in plenty of boiling water for about 35 minutes. Peel the potatoes and press them through a potato press into a bowl.

4. Prick the dough base several times with a fork. Cover the base with a suitable piece of baking paper and place dried legumes on top for blind baking. Slide the oven shelf onto the bottom of the oven. Bake the base of the dough in the preheated oven at 180°C (convection 160°C, gas: level 2–3) on the oven rack for 15 minutes, remove.

5. Remove the pulses and paper and bake the base for 5 minutes.

6. Mix sweet potatoes with eggs, whipped cream, the remaining whole cane sugar, maple syrup and cinnamon.

7. Place the sweet potato mixture on the pre-baked base and bake at 180°C (fan oven 160°C, gas: level 2–3) on the second rack from the bottom for 40–45 minutes until the mixture has thickened. Let cool on an oven rack before serving.

Nutritional value

- 389 calories
- Protein 4.5g
- Carbohydrates 47.8g
- Fat 20.6g
- Cholesterol 78.2mg
- Sodium 253.7mg

Sweet Pumpkin Buns

Total Time 2 h 55 min

Serving 8

Ingredients

- 300 grams Hokkaido pumpkin

- 50 milliliters orange juice

- 450 g spelled flour type 1050

- 1 cube yeast

- 70 grams whole cane sugar

- 150 milliliters lukewarm milk (3.5% fat)

- 1 vanilla pod

- 1 egg (m)

- 80 grams butter at room temperature

- ½ teaspoon cinnamon

- 1 pinch cardamom powder

- 1 pinch salt

- 1 egg yolk

Preparation

1. Wash the pumpkin, core it and dice it. Put the orange juice in a saucepan and cook over low heat until soft, about 15 minutes.

2. Let the purée and cool.

3. Meanwhile, in a bowl, put the flour and make a well in the middle. Crumble the yeast and add 1 teaspoon of sugar and milk to the hollow of the whole cane. Cover for 10 minutes and let rise.

4. Slit the lengthwise vanilla pod and scrape the pulp out. The vanilla pulp, the remaining sugar, egg, butter, cinnamon, cardamom, a pinch of salt and the cooled pumpkin puree are added to the pre-dough. Knead and cover everything to smooth the dough and let it rise for 1 hour.

5. Divide the dough into 8 pieces of equal shape and form into rolls. Place it on a baking sheet lined with paper for baking. With water, whisk the egg yolks and brush the rolls with them.

6. Bake the rolls at 180°C (convection 160°C, gas: level 2–3) in a preheated oven for 20–30 minutes until they are golden brown.

Nutritional value

- **Net carbohydrates:** 1% (1g)

- **Fiber:** 0g

- **Fat:** 85% (31g)

- **Protein:** 14% (11g)

- **Kcal:** 327

Steamed Vegetables and Fried Tofu

Total time 50mins

Serving 4

Ingredients

- 4 carrots
- 8 baby pak choi
- 20 grams ginger
- 100 milliliters vegetable broth
- 2 tablespoon sweet chili sauce
- 2 tablespoon rice wine
- 1 lime juice
- 1 shallot
- 4 tablespoon soybean oil
- 80 milliliters teriyaki sauce
- 600 grams tofu
- 3 tablespoon chickpea flour

Preparation

1. Peel the carrots and quarter them lengthways. Wash the pak choi, cut in half and place in a steamer basket. Peel and dice the ginger. Sprinkle on the pak choi and steam in a closed pan for 5–6 minutes.

2. Heat the vegetable stock, stir in the chilli sauce, rice wine and limes. Place the finished pak choi in a bowl, drizzle with the stock and let it stand covered.

3. Peel the shallot, dice it finely and sauté it in 1 tablespoon of hot oil. Deglaze with the teriyaki sauce and simmer a little, then remove from the heat.

4. Cut the tofu into slices and turn in the chickpea flour. Heat a tablespoon of oil in a wok and fry the carrots for 3–4 minutes over a medium temperature. Then take it out and add to the pak choi. Heat the remaining oil in the wok and fry the tofu on both sides until light brown. Arrange on the vegetables and serve drizzled with the teriyaki sauce.

Nutritional value

- **Calories 83 kcal / 100gr**

- **Protein 8 gr / 100gr**

- **Fat 4.7 gr / 100gr**

- **Carbohydrates 1.8 gr / 100gr**

BBQ Pulled Sweet Potato Burger

Total time 1hr

Serving 4

Ingredients

For the quick BBQ sauce

- 400 milliliters tomatoes

- 1 tablespoon tomato paste

- 1 garlic

- 1 teaspoon olive oil

- 2 tablespoons soy sauce

- 1 tablespoon rice syrup

- 2 teaspoon paprika powder (smoked)

- 1 teaspoon garam masala

- Salt and pepper

For the BBQ Pulled Sweet Potato

- 800 grams sweet potatoes

- Salt

- 2 tablespoons olive oil

- 1 onion

For the peanut cream

- 100 milliliters peanut oil

- 100 milliliters soy drink (soy milk)

- 1 teaspoon mustard

- 2 tablespoons apple cider vinegar

- Salt

- 2 tablespoons peanut butter

For the eggplant bacon

- 8 slices eggplant

- 4 tablespoons soy sauce

- 1 tablespoon paprika powder (smoked)

- 2 teaspoon rice syrup

For the BBQ Pulled Sweet Potato Burger

- 4 buns

- 8 simply v gourmet slices spicy

- 8 slices cucumber

- 1 Coriander (chopped)

- 6 tablespoons peanut butter

- 4 tablespoons peanut kernel (chopped)

Preparation

1. Mix all the ingredients for the quick BBQ sauce.

2. For the BBQ Pulled Sweet Potato, peel the sweet potatoes, cut into approx. 0.5 cm thick slices and then cut each of them into fine strips. Peel the onion, and then dice it finely.

3. Heat the olive oil in a pan, then add the sweet potato strips and the onion cubes, season with salt and sauté over medium heat for about 5 minutes.

4. Reduce the heat, add the sauce to the pan and stir in, allow reducing. If the sweet potato strips are still too firm, add some water to the pan and reduce it again. If necessary, repeat the process until the sweet potato strips have reached the desired firm consistency.

5. For the peanut cream, put all the ingredients except for the puree in a blender and let it become a cream. Add the peanut butter, stir.

6. For the eggplant bacon, preheat the oven to 200 degrees. Place the eggplant in a baking dish. Mix the soy sauce, paprika powder and rice syrup, then pour over the eggplant.

7. Put the baking pan in the oven, bake for about 20–25 minutes until the eggplant has taken on color. Remove and drain on a kitchen towel.

8. Place the baby leaves, cucumber slices and BBQ pulled sweet potato and eggplant bacon on top, sprinkle with coriander. Brush the top with peanut cream and sprinkle with chopped peanuts. Put both sides together and enjoy.

Nutritional value

- Calories 985 kcal (47%)

- Protein 25 g (26%)

- Fat 56 g (48%)

- Carbohydrates 94 g (63%)

- Added sugar 7 g (28%)

- Fiber 15.4 g (51%)

Chapter Ten:
Keto Diet Meal Plan

Day 1

- **Breakfast:** Scrambled eggs with sautéed onion and cheddar cheese.

- **Snack:** Peanut butter caramel crunchy bar.

- **Lunch:** 150g ham, 2 cups mixed greens with ½ avocado, 5 large black olives, ½ cup sliced cucumbers, and 2 tablespoons blue cheese vinaigrette.

- **Snack:** 3/4 medium zucchini cut into sticks and 80g provolone.

- **Dinner:** Baked catfish with broccoli and herb butter mix.

Day 2

- **Breakfast:** fluffy omelette.

- **Mid-morning:** a fresh half-orange and a handful of sunflower seeds.

- **Food:** baked chicken breasts with morbier cheese.

- **Snack:** natural unsweetened yogurt with chia seeds.

- **Dinner:** baked salmon with nuts.

Day 3

- **Breakfast** avocados with baked eggs

- **Mid-morning** roasted pumpkin seeds or seeds.

- **Food** roast beef round with boiled eggs. Half peach

- **Snack** natural unsweetened yogurt with chopped almonds.

- **Dinner** Turkish eggs with yogurt.

Day 4

- **Breakfast:** cloud bread or cloud bread with fresh cheese.

- **Mid-morning:** a handful of nuts.

- **Food:** juicy chicken breast baked with 50 grams of lettuce with olive oil.

- **Snack:** creamy chocolate and avocado.

- **Dinner:** a cod omelette.

Day 5

- **Breakfast:** eggs in a serrano ham casserole.

- **Mid-morning:** natural unsweetened yogurt with sunflower seeds.

- **Food:** baked salmon with garlic sauce.

- **Snack:** sugar-free cheesecake with one or two strawberries only.

- **Dinner:** baked avocados stuffed with salmon and egg.

Day 6

- **Breakfast:** Scrambled eggs with sautéed onion and cheddar cheese.

- **Snack:** Peanut butter caramel crunchy bar.

- **Lunch: 150g** ham, 2 cups mixed greens with ½ avocado, 5 large black olives, ½ cup sliced cucumbers, and 2 tablespoons blue cheese vinaigrette.

- **Snack:** 3/4 medium zucchini cut into sticks and 80g provolone.

- **Dinner:** baked catfish with broccoli and herb butter mix.

Day 7

- **Breakfast:** quick omelette with fresh herbs.

- **Mid-morning:** natural unsweetened yogurt with chopped almonds.

- **Food:** poached eggs with gulas and prawns. Half apricot

- **Snack:** tea or coffee without sugar and panna cotta with cocoa.

- **Dinner:** eggs on the plate with sobrasada.

Day 8

- **Breakfast**: two fried eggs in served butter with greens sautéed grazed.

- **Lunch:** A bunless grass-fed hamburger garnished with cheese, mushrooms, and avocado on a bed of green vegetables.

- **Dinner:** Pork chops with green beans sautéed in coconut oil.

Day 9

- **Breakfast**: a mushroom omelet.

- **Lunch:** tuna salad with celery and tomato on a bed of green vegetables.

- **Dinner:** roasted chicken with cream sauce and broccoli sautéed.

Day 10

- **Breakfast**: peppers stuffed with cheese and eggs.

- **Lunch:** arugula salad with boiled eggs, turkey, avocado, and blue cheese.

- **Dinner:** grilled salmon with spinach sautéed in coconut oil.

Day 11

- **Breakfast**: fat yogurt topped with granola full Keto.

- **Lunch:** Steak bowl with cauliflower rice, cheese, herbs, avocado, and salsa.

- **Dinner:** bison steak with cheesy broccoli.

Day 12

- **Breakfast:** avocado Egg boat oven.

- **Lunch:** Caesar salad with chicken.

- **Dinner:** pork chops with vegetables.

Day 13

- **Breakfast**: toast Chou-flower topped with cheese and avocado.

- **Lunch:** Salmon burgers with bun-less pesto topped.

- **Dinner:** meatballs served with zucchini noodles and parmesan cheese.

Day 14

- **Breakfast**: coconut milk pudding with chia garnished with coconut and nuts.

- **Lunch:** Cobb salad with vegetables, boiled eggs, avocado, cheese, and turkey.

- **Dinner:** chicken with coconut curry.

Day 15

- **Breakfast:** Scrambled eggs with sautéed onion and cheddar cheese.

- **Snack:** Peanut butter caramel crunchy bar.

- **Lunch:** 150g ham, 2 cups mixed greens with ½ avocado, 5 large black olives, ½ cup sliced cucumbers, and 2 tablespoons blue cheese vinaigrette.

- **Snack:** 3/4 medium zucchini cut into sticks and 80g provolone.

- **Dinner:** Baked catfish with broccoli and herb butter mix.

Day 16

- **Breakfast**: Scrambled eggs with sautéed onion and cheddar cheese.

- **Snack:** 1 cup sliced red bell pepper with 2 tablespoons ranch dressing.

- **Lunch:** Bacon cheddar soup.

- **Snack:** 1 stalk of celery with 2 tablespoons of cream cheese.

- **Dinner:** Bone-in pork chop and 300 grams of cauliflower and cheddar puree.

Day 17

- **Breakfast**: Spinach and Swiss cheese omelette.

- **Snack:** An Iso Whey Zero and Omega 3 protein shake.

- **Lunch:** Grilled chicken with baby spinach, tomato, and avocado salad.

- **Snack:** 80g of ham, 2 tablespoons of cream cheese and 2 pieces of pickles.

- **Dinner:** Sautéed beef with vegetables in a romaine salad.

Day 18

- **Breakfast:** Cheese and spinach omelette with avocado and salsa.

- **Snack:** An Iso Whey Zero and Omega 3 protein shake.

- **Lunch:** Chicken tart with a green salad.

- **Snack:** ½ medium zucchini cut into sticks and 40 grams of cheese of your choice.

- **Dinner:** 250g of hamburger with 40g of pepper cheese, 1 small tomato, ½ avocado, and 2 leaves of romaine lettuce.

Day 19

- **Breakfast:** 2 large eggs, ¼ cup grated cheddar cheese, and 4 tablespoons raw salsa or pico de gallo.

- **Snack**: An Iso Whey Zero and Omega 3 protein shake.

- **Lunch**: Chili con carne with 2 cups of mixed vegetables, and 2 tablespoons of Italian vinaigrette.

- **Snack**: 1 cup sliced red bell pepper with 2 tablespoons ranch dressing.

- **Dinner (6g net carbs):** Caesar salad without croutons.

Day 20

- **Breakfast:** Red pepper stuffed with creamy eggs and spinach.

- **Snack:** An Iso Whey Zero and Omega 3 protein shake.

- **Lunch:** Tuna salad with 170 grams of tuna, 2 stalks of celery, 1 pickled gherkin, 2 tablespoons of mayonnaise.

- **Snack:** 1 portobello mushroom, ¼-cup raw sauce and 40 grams of pepper cheese.

- **Dinner:** 200 grams of Italian sausage, ¼ medium onion sliced, ½-sliced red bell pepper with 2 cups of spinach, ½ cup of sliced mushrooms, and 2 tablespoons of blue cheese vinaigrette.

Day 21

- **Breakfast:** Flaxseed and pumpkin pancakes.

- **Snack:** 5 whole peas and 80g cheddar cheese.

- **Lunch:** 250 grams of chicken breast in 2 cups of romaine lettuce, with 5 radishes, and 2 tablespoons of creamy Italian dressing.

- **Snack:** 2 celery stalks and 2 tablespoons cream cheese.

- **Dinner:** Baked salmon with chermoula on broccoli.

Day 22

- **Breakfast:** an omelette of two eggs with spinach and mushrooms with coconut oil.

- **Snack:** a handful of blueberries.

- **Lunch:** salad with chicken, artichokes, tomatoes, herbs, egg, and olive oil.

- **Dinner:** baked salmon and green salad with avocado and olive oil.

Day 23

- **Breakfast:** two eggs fried in olive oil and 1/2 avocado with tomatoes and cilantro.

- **Snack:** a piece of soft cheese with cucumber slices.

- **Lunch:** bacon and tomatoes on bread.

- **Dinner:** ground beef and homemade tomato sauce.

Day 24

- **Breakfast:** bacon and eggs.

- **Snack:** a handful of almonds.

- **Lunch:** roast beef, arugula, pesto, and olive oil.

- **Dinner:** shrimp, tomato and avocado salad with olive oil and lime.

Day 25

- **Breakfast:** omelet with broccoli.

- **Snack:** celery and peanut butter.

- **Lunch:** slices of turkey, almonds, avocado, cucumber, and a handful of blueberries.

- **Dinner:** lamb ribs with herbal oil.

Day 26

- **Breakfast:** scrambled eggs in butter with tomatoes and cilantro.

- **Snack:** green peppers with cream cheese.

- **Lunch:** salami, soft cheese, radish, avocado, and olive oil.

- **Dinner:** chicken salad with tomatoes.

Day 27

- **Breakfast:** boiled eggs.

- **Snack:** bacon and lettuce.

- **Lunch:** chicken salad with olive oil.

- **Dinner:** baked chicken and cabbage.

Day 28

- **Breakfast:** eggplants fried in olive oil with eggs.

- **Snack:** homemade zucchini chips.

- **Lunch:** salami, roasted peppers, and green salad.

- **Dinner:** baked salmon with pesto and Brussels sprouts.

Day 29

- **Breakfast: a** fluffy omelette.

- **Mid-morning:** a fresh half-orange and a handful of sunflower seeds.

- **Food:** baked chicken breasts with morbier cheese.

- **Snack:** natural unsweetened yogurt with chia seeds.

- **Dinner:** baked salmon with nuts.

Day 30

- **Breakfast:** avocados with baked eggs.

- **Mid-morning:** roasted pumpkin seeds or seeds.

- **Food:** roast beef round with boiled eggs. Half peach.

- **Snack:** natural unsweetened yogurt with chopped almonds.

- **Dinner:** Turkish eggs with yogurt.

KETO FOR WOMEN OVER 50

CONCLUSION

The ketogenic diet is not for everyone, just for people who want to enjoy a better lifestyle, reaping more benefits such as improved mental performance and increased fat burning as a source of energy.

Now that you know the benefits of ketosis, we recommend taking a cup of fasting Super Coffee in the morning and fasting until lunchtime. This will help you get into ketosis even if you are not on a low carbohydrate diet.

Made in the USA
Monee, IL
08 August 2021